A Medical Doctor's Guide to YOUTH, HEALTH, AND LONGEVITY

A Medical Doctor's Guide to YOUTH, HEALTH, AND LONGEVITY

John Deaton, M.D.

Parker Publishing Company, Inc.

West Nyack, New York

Library of Congress Cataloging in Publication Data

Deaton, John G
    A medical doctor's guide to youth, health, and
longevity.

    Includes index.
        1. Health. 2. Medicine, Popular. I. Title.
II. Title: Youth, health, and longevity. [DNLM:
1. Hygiene. 2. Mental health. QT180 D284m]
RA776.5.D38   613   77-3385
ISBN 0-13-572503-8

To Helen and Gilbert Garrett,
and
to Janet and Kenneth Ragsdale

muchas gracias

What This Book

Can Do for You

Doctors learn to expect questions from other people. The question I am most often asked is not about disease but about health. It is, "What can I do to feel better?"

People want to know how to feel their very best every day. They want their minds and bodies to be vigorous and youthful. They want to know how to lose weight and how to get to sleep the natural way. They want to know how to treat their aching feet, their arthritis and their blood pressure. They want to know how to prevent indigestion and gas, what to do for headache, sunburn, rash, tired eyes, sinus, constipation, backache and many other things. They ask advice because they want to live their lives to the fullest. They want to enjoy the best health possible.

You, too, can enjoy the best health possible. You can do this by applying the knowledge in this book to your own life.

Your Right to Health and Happiness

Like life, liberty and the pursuit of happiness, health is your inherent right. Unfortunately, it is not protected by law—not completely. True, immunizations have just about wiped out some killer diseases of old, such as smallpox and polio, but conditions such as arthritis and high blood pressure and heart disease are as common as ever. There is much you can do *on your own* to improve or prevent these problems. Further, you can take care of yourself when minor illness arrives and get back on your feet that much quicker! Improving your health can reap benefits financially. You may be able to get by with less medicine and fewer trips to the physician. Finally, by following the advice in this book you will feel better every day, and you will add extra years to your life. The best thing of all is that *good health will enable you to live life to its fullest!* Yes, a healthy body is your inherent right, and you can cash in on this right by applying to your own life the chapter-by-chapter information given in this book.

How You Benefit from Healthy Living

We live in the day of the medical miracle. Antibiotics can easily wipe out germs that used to cause serious infections, and even miraculous procedures such as transplantation of the human kidney are coming to be a part of ordinary medical care. But doctors can't do everything. They cannot do your healthy living for you.

You can benefit from *A Medical Doctor's Guide to Youth, Health, and Longevity,* but only if you apply to your own life this information that has helped so many others. Your individual health is determined by many things. One of the most important, though, is what you choose to do for yourself. You treat your health every time you sit down to eat, every time you exercise or don't exercise, every time you do something that is good for you. This book, by showing the things you can do to enjoy better health, will help you to realize your greatest health potential. It will help you to feel better.

The Health-Giving Promise of This Book

This book is an outgrowth of my years of training and professional experience in practicing medicine and in answering those questions I mentioned earlier. Like many physicians, I have come to realize that the practical lessons of experience have been as helpful to me as the formal training I had years ago in medical school. Practical, easy-to-understand health tips are what fill this book. If you choose to use them you can enjoy youth, health and longevity. That's my promise to you.

John Deaton, M.D.

Author's Note

The case histories in this book serve as illustrations of how various people have enjoyed better health from following the information laid down in the step-by-step directions. Patients I have treated should not look for themselves too closely in these case histories. I respect the right of everyone to privacy and for this reason have changed names, joggled times and identities and in several instances drawn a composite patient to illustrate a point. Some of the case histories were taken from medical articles I have read, and still others represent persons I have been told about by other physicians or health workers.

Contents

What This Book Can Do for You 5

Author's Note 7

1. Building Rich Red Blood for Better Health 19

Five Tips on How to Increase Your Blood Count
(19) . . . How Charlene Raised Her Blood Count and Cured
Her Fatigue at the Same Time (20) . . . Getting All the Iron
You Need from What You Eat (21) . . . The Magical Effects
That Iron Has in the Bloodstream (21) . . . The Man Who
Drank So Much That His Blood Turned to Water
(22) . . . The Importance of Eating to Build the Blood in
Every Way (23) . . . How Mary S. Solved Her Iron-Deficiency
the Effortless Way (23) . . . Getting at the Bottom of Blood
Loss (24) . . . The Man Who Won the Battle but Lost the War
(24) . . . Some Things to Watch for (25) . . . When Taking
Iron Tablets Can Be Helpful (26) . . . Avoiding Blood-
Damaging Chemicals (26) . . . The Woman Who Learned the
Hard Way That Drugs Can Be Bad as Well as Good
(27) . . . How Adelle Turned a Simple Treatment into a
Blood-Building Process (28) . . . Taking Advantage of the
Fact That Clearing Up Disease in One Part of Your Body
Can Help the Rest of You (29) . . . The Neglected Ingredient
You Can Use to Build Rich Red Blood (29) . . . A Trick You
Can Learn from the Athletes (29)

2. Deriving Energy from the Things That Used to
Make You Tired 31

Mae's Discovery of a Quick Way to Have Energy in Abun-
dance (31) . . . Taking Advantage of Three Quick Sources of
Energy (32) . . . How to Have Power in Reserve
(33) . . . Learning to Draw Power from Natural Sources
(34) . . . The Man Who Discovered That Exercise Is Better
Than Any Drug (35) . . . Three Ways to Make Pepping Up a

Habit (36) . . . The Woman Who Reshaped Her Life by
Reshaping Her Body (36) . . . Accomplishing Many Things
by Doing One (37) . . . Ed S.'s Remedy for Insomnia and
Fatigue (38) . . . Why the Natural Way Is the Best Way
(38) . . . The Girl Who Took Too Many (39) . . . How to Fill
Your Life with the Energy That Comes from Natural Sleep
(39) . . . Getting the Rest You Need (41)

3.   **How to Have Better Health from What You Eat** **42**

What You Eat Does Make a Difference (42) . . . Seven Tips to
Save You Money and Improve Your Health (43) . . . How Ed
S. Got Each Day Started the Right Way with a Healthy
Breakfast (44) . . . The Energy for Your Day Doesn't Come
from What You Eat for Breakfast (44) . . . Raymond's
Discovery of a Diet That Prevented His Attacks of Joint Pain
(46) . . . Taking Advantage of Martha's "Magic" Cure for
Diabetes (48) . . . Diseases That Eating Right Can Prevent or
"Cure" (49) . . . Food Allergies and How to Prevent Them
(50) . . . Rosalind's Discovery of How to Prevent Skin Rash
(50) . . . How Thurmond Overcame His Attacks of Diarrhea
(50) . . . Let Your Symptoms Be Your Guide (51) . . . The
Elimination Diet (51)

4.   **Taking Advantage of the Natural Ways
to Control Your Blood Pressure** **53**

How Tom Learned to Lower His Blood Pressure without
Drugs (53) . . . Avoiding Something That Can Sneak Up on
You (54) . . . Blood Pressure Drugs Work by Eliminating Salt
from the Body (55) . . . Putting an Ill-Advised Habit Behind
You (55) . . . How Katie W. Learned about Salt Intake the
Hard Way (57) . . . The Physician Who Learned of an Active,
Drugless Way to Lower Blood Pressure (58) . . . How Exer-
cise Brings the Blood Pressure Down (59) . . . Deriving Max-
imum Benefit from Your Own Acitivities (59) . . . The Thing
That Made All the Difference in Reducing Earlene's Blood
Pressure (60) . . . Five Steps to Developing Your Own Blood-
Pressure-Lowering Activity (62) . . . How Mrs. B. Learned
That Personal Exercise Is Easy Exercise (62) . . . How George
Learned an Important Blood-Pressure-Lowering Secret
(65) . . . Taking the Time to Handle Stress in a Healthy Man-
ner (66) . . . How Eldon Gave Up One Thing and Got Two
Things in Return (67) . . . The Single Act That Can Mean So

Much (68) . . . Probably the Most Important Thing You Can Do (68) . . . How All These Things Work Together to Help You (68) . . . Knowing When Your Pressure Is Normal and When It Isn't (69) . . . How to Take Your Own Blood Pressure (69)

5. **Boosting Your Vitality by Keeping Your Heart and Vessels Young** 71

The Day Jack C. Learned the Truth about Heart Disease (71) . . . The Most Important Lesson Is the Easiest One to Forget (73) . . . How the Healthy Way to a Man's Heart Can Be through His Stomach (73) . . . How Lonnie Learned to Start the Day the Right Way (76) . . . What You Hear May Not Necessarily Be True (77) . . . How Sherry Learned the Benefits of a Cereal Breakfast (78) . . . The Man Who Turned Sensible Eating to His Advantage in His Fight against Heart Disease (80) . . . Taking Advantage of the Two Body Parts Brenda Used in Her Winning Fight against Heart Failure (81) . . . How You Benefit from Keeping the World's Most Fantastic Pump in Tip-Top Shape (82) . . . How Bob Discovered the Right Way and the Wrong Way to Exercise (83) . . . Making the Best Use of Your Own Program (84) . . . The Ninety-Year-Old Man Who Wants to Die Running (85) . . . How You Can Exercise in Spite of Medical Problems (85) . . . How Rudy M. Learned That Smoking Does Have an Effect on the Heart (86) . . . Protecting Yourself from This Silent Killer (86) . . . Learning to Boost Your Heart Function by Conserving Your Energy (87)

6. **Staying Young by Losing Pounds the Natural Way** 88

How Joanna Learned the Truth about Weight Loss (88) . . . Taking Advantage of Three Ways to Slim Down and Stay that Way (89) . . . The Truth about Calories (89) . . . Seven Tips You Can Use to Stay Young by Losing Pounds the Natural Way (90) . . . How Shelton N. Discovered One Thing about Himself—and Lost 50 Pounds (91) . . . The Way George Avoided Eating Food That He Didn't Need (92) . . . The Way Helen Used Her Talents to Lose Weight Instead of Gaining It (94) . . . The Six-Feedings Diet (95) . . . Vanessa's Discovery of Calorie Burning and How She Used It to Lose Fifteen Pounds (96) . . . The Way to

Eat and Still Lose Weight (97) . . . Try this Twenty-Minute Refresher (98) . . . The Secret of Youth Is as Near as the Street (99) . . . How Norman Learned to Set Realistic Goals—and Achieve Them (99) . . . How to Be Your Own Best Friend (100)

7. **Making Use of Home Treatments to Relieve the
    Pain and Stiffness of Arthritis** **101**

Choosing One of Five Methods to Treat Arthritis (101) . . . How Sally D. Caught On to a Little-Known Way to Treat Arthritis (102) . . . Five Ways to Use Heat to Relieve Pain and Stiffness (102) . . . The Benefits You Can Expect (105) . . . How Maxine Z. Learned to Keep Her Hands and Shoulders Free from Stiffness (105) . . . Getting Full Movement in Spite of Arthritis (106) . . . The Exercises to Perform (107) . . . What Exercise Will Do for You (108) . . . The Importance of Body Movement (109) . . . Giving Your Body What It Needs (109) . . . Choosing What Works Best for You (110) . . . Six Ways to Take Advantage of Gravity (111) . . . Using the One Drug That Helps the Most (112) . . . How Merrill Learned the Truth about Pain Relievers (112) . . . Two Things That Can Make All the Difference in Your Winning Fight against Arthritis (114) . . . The Decision That Changed Ramona's Life (115)

8. **Keeping Your Kidneys Fit by Using the
    Least Expensive Medicine in the World** **117**

How Etta B. Learned That the Least Expensive Medicines Are Often the Best (117) . . . Putting the Least Expensive Medicine to Work for You (118) . . . The Natural Way Joe Discovered to Avoid Kidney Stones (119) . . . Using Three Natural Antiseptics That Help to Cleanse the Urinary Tract (120) . . . Jane's Discovery of an Overlooked Way to Protect Her Bladder and Kidneys (120) . . . The Man Who Drank His Medicine Three Times a Day (121) . . . A Good Practice for Anyone Who Desires Good Health (122) . . . The Diet That Can Take a Load off the Kidneys (123) . . . Eating Right to Avoid the Symptoms of Disease (124)

9. **Natural Ways to Keep Your Digestive Tract
    Healthy and Comfortable** **126**

How Jean A. Kicked the Laxative Habit by Using the Best

Medicine of All (126) . . . Drinking Your Way to the Healthy, Natural Rhythm (128) . . . The Advantages of Doing Things the Regular Way (128) . . . Enjoying the Benefits of Food Laxatives (129) . . . How Royce Discovered That One Thing Can Make All the Difference in Having Normal Bowel Movements or Being Constipated (129) . . . Taking Full Advantage of Body Movement (130) . . . How Ruth C. Got Relief from Gas and Heartburn by Using a Safe and Simple Remedy (130) . . . Four Ways to Overcome Peptic Esophagitis (131) . . . Choosing the Antacid Therapy That Is Right for You (132) . . . The Best Way to Control an Ulcer (133) . . . The Thing John B. Did to Cure His Ulcer (133) . . . Three Ways to Have a Healthier Stomach (134) . . . The Painless Way of Warding Off Attacks of "Colitis" (135) . . . How Wesley Learned to Avoid His Attacks of Diarrhea (135) . . . Natural Ways to Treat Diarrhea (136)

10. **Keeping Your Skin Young and Alive
    by Using Natural Remedies** 137

Fay's Discovery of a Way to Keep Her Skin Young (138) . . . Putting Fay's Method to Work for You (139) . . . How Vicki Relieved the Itching and Flaking of Dry Skin (139) . . . Three Ways to Relieve the Symptoms of Dry Skin (140) . . . How Lareina Learned That Natural Skin Care is the Best Skin Care (141) . . . How to Avoid the Things That Harm Your Skin (141) . . . The Trick Homer R. Used to Keep from Getting Poison Ivy (142) . . . How to Save Yourself Two Weeks of Itching (142) . . . What to Do When Itching Does Occur (143) . . . Choosing Your Skin Care as You Eat (144) . . . The Man Who Took Something for Headache and Ended Up in the Hospital (145) . . . Keeping Away from Drugs That Can Harm You (145)

11. **Natural Ways That Will Free You from Headache** 147

How Sylvia Got Relief by Getting to the Bottom of Her Problem (141) . . . Finding the Cause Is the First Step to Curing the Headache (148) . . . Putting Your New Knowledge to Work for You (149) . . . How Bob B. Solved His Headache Problem in an Unexpected Way (150) . . . Getting Relief from Breaking the Routine (151) . . . How Vera J. Made Use of a Little-Known Prescription for Headache (152) . . . An Easy

Method Barbara Used to Have Fewer Migraine Headaches
(153) . . . Taking the Logical Approach to Migraine
(153) . . . Separating the Minor Headache from the One That
Could Be Serious (154) . . . What Medicine to Use and How
to Use It (155)

12. How to Do Your Feet a Favor **156**

How Clara M. Made One Change and Never Regretted It
(156) . . . Some Little-Known Tips You Can Use in Buying
Footwear (157) . . . How Howard Learned to Reinvigorate
His Feet (158) . . . The Delightful Way to Enliven Your Feet
(159) . . . How to Take the Biggest Load off Your Feet
(159) . . . How Peggy W. Got Relief of Swelling by
Eliminating One Thing from Her Diet (160) . . . The Benefits
of Using Madge T.'s Method to Control Varicose Veins
(160) . . . How to Give Your Feet the Conditioning They
Need (161) . . . Common Sense Ways to Treat Common Foot
Problems (161)

13. Home Remedies for Some Common Problems **164**

Rodney's Solution to His Bad Back Problem (164) . . . Four
Steps to Overcoming Backache (165) . . . The Man Who
Treated His Backache by Sleeping at the Office (166) . . . How
to Firm Up Your Own Bed (167) . . . What to Do When You
Have Fever (168) . . . Cynthia's Method of Relieving Mild
Fever (168) . . . Relieving Mild Fever with the Best Treatment
Possible (169) . . . Common Sense for the Common Cold and
Flu (169) . . . Chasing a Cold Away When You Get One
(170) . . . Three Ways to Overcome Nagging Mouth Ulcers
(171)

14. How to Look and Feel Your Best Every Day **173**

Harry O.'s Secret for Sales Success (173) . . . Try This One-
Minute Pause That Can Refresh and Invigorate You
(174) . . . How Liz Did One Thing and Changed Her Entire
Life (175) . . . Taking Your Place in the World by Speaking
Your Own Mind (176) . . . The Woman Whose Courage
Changed a Cloud of Smoke to Clean, Fresh Air
(177) . . . Solving Problems by Talking Them Out with
Someone Else (177) . . . Darlene's Discovery of a Way to Be
Happy (177) . . . How to Fill Your Life with Happy Things

(179) . . . The Clean-Living Way to a Long and Happy Life
(180) . . . To Your Good Health and Longevity (181)

Desirable Weights for Adult Women 182

Desirable Weights for Adult Men 183

Index 185

A Medical Doctor's Guide to
YOUTH, HEALTH,
AND LONGEVITY

1

Building Rich Red Blood for Better Health

Everyone wants to have rich red blood! Long before men understood this precious fluid, they equated it with health and youth and vigor. Roman spectators used to rush into the arena to drink the blood of a just-killed gladiator. During the middle ages the drinking of blood was a remedy for certain diseases, and it is said that in 1492 three young boys were sacrificed so that their blood could be given to the ailing Pope Innocent VIII. Only a few years ago traveling "medicine men" could easily hawk their alcoholic medicinals by claiming that the tonic "built up the blood." Even today, products such as Geritol are bought and consumed by people who want a blood-building tonic.

You can have rich blood and enjoy better health from it. However, in all likelihood you don't need a medicine to strengthen your blood. What you need are some natural blood-building activities. Here are five ways to have rich red blood:

Five Tips on How to Increase Your Blood Count

1. *Eat foods that build the blood.*
2. *Check any sources of blood loss.*
3. *Avoid blood-damaging chemicals.*
4. *Make sure any chronic infection is cleared up.*
5. *Exercise regularly.*

The simple truth about blood is this. The people who have the richest, reddest blood are the same people who have the healthiest hearts, lungs, kidneys and livers. In other words, they are people who are healthy. Good health is a product of many things, and it starts with eating foods that will help your body make rich, robust red blood cells.

How Charlene Raised Her Blood Count and Cured Her Fatigue at the Same Time

Charlene was a 60-year-old widow who lived alone. She came to me in a roundabout way. Her cat got out of her apartment and climbed a tree across the street. A neighborhood boy climbed the tree and returned the pet, but the child cut his leg on a sharp branch. Charlene brought him to have the cut bandaged, and while talking to her I realized she looked anemic.

"As a matter of fact," she said, "I feel tired, doctor. Not too many years ago I could have climbed that tree to get Chester back. I guess I'm just getting old."

"Maybe and maybe not. Why don't we get a blood test and see?" While the technician was doing the blood count, I examined Charlene and took her medical history. Her physical examination was normal, and she had no history of blood loss. What she did admit to was a diet that I immediately recognized was deficient in iron.

"I don't cook for anyone but myself, and I'm afraid that much of the time I don't cook at all. I open a can of soup for supper and get by on a few fruits and vegetables the rest of the day. I eat a lot of potatoes. Do they contain iron?"

I told her that potatoes contained some iron, that most foods have at least a small amount of iron. But the foods that are richest in iron—lean red meat, liver and iron-enriched flour products—were the very ones she wasn't eating. Three months after Charlene changed her eating habits her red blood count was much improved, and it rose to normal during the ensuing months. But the biggest surprise was in how Charlene felt.

"I was in a rut and didn't realize how dead tired I was until I began to feel better. Doctor, I'm not old! I'm young! I feel great! I've got a niece in San Francisco who's been trying for years to get me to come see her, and I'm going. But don't worry. I'll keep eating right even after I get to California."

Getting All the Iron You Need from What You Eat

Iron deficiency is probably the most common form of anemia in the world. This is paradoxical when you consider the abundant supplies of iron in the earth's crust, but to enter the human body the iron must first get into the food that we eat. Thus, the foods you set on your table actually determine whether or not you will have rich red blood.

Here is a partial list of the foods that are richest in iron. Select the ones you like the best and put them into your menu every day!

- *Lean red meat.* This is the best source of dietary iron. Lean red meat means steak, veal cutlets, hamburger meat, roast, lamb, chicken and ham. To build healthy blood, you need two helpings of meat a day.

- *Liver.* Liver is an excellent source of dietary iron. If you are one of the lucky people who enjoys eating liver, you can add variety to your diet by eating it once or twice a week.

- *Iron-enriched flour products.* By law, most breads are made from iron-enriched flour. Choose these products in preference to non-enriched ones. Keep in mind that whole wheat or whole rye bread is generally a better source of iron and other nutrients than processed (white) bread.

- *Whole grain cereals.* These are good sources of iron. Some people add extra iron enrichment to their cereal by sprinkling it with wheat germ.

- *Eggs.* Egg yolks are rich in iron. Unfortunately, egg yolks also contain a lot of cholesterol and saturated fats, and for this reason are not good for your heart. However, it is all right to eat eggs on a short-term basis when you need to build your blood back up if it has become deficient in iron.

The Magical Effects That Iron Has in the Bloodstream

A good intake of dietary iron is one of the best ways you can build rich red blood. The reason for iron's importance is that it is the element in the red blood cell that carries oxygen from the lungs to the rest of the body. Blood containing lots of oxygen looks rich and red, while blood that contains little oxygen has a dull, dark appearance. Without iron, blood cells cannot form normally. The blood count drops, the blood becomes thin, and it loses its power. The condition is known as anemia.

Iron deficiency is the most common cause of anemia, but the body also needs other nutrients to build healthy blood. What can happen to the blood when it doesn't get these nutrients is shown by the case of

The Man Who Drank So Much That His Blood Turned to Water

Walter H. was an alcoholic, and he didn't come to the emergency room seeking medical help. He was brought in by a policeman who had arrested him for disturbing the peace. Walter was having trouble getting his breath, and the policeman decided to have him checked by a physician before taking him to jail. That decision saved Walter's life.

He was suffering from pulmonary edema, a deadly condition of lung failure, and it was all he could do to move air in and out of his water-logged lungs. The cause of the pulmonary edema was an extremely low blood count. In fact, the laboratory technician who called me in the emergency room to report the results of the blood test said, "What's this guy been drinking? His blood has turned to water."

Of course, most of the blood is water even in a healthy person. What the technician meant was that Walter's red blood cell count was extremely low. He had the worst case of anemia I've ever seen.

Walter could breathe much easier after several blood transfusions. The day after his admission to the hospital he told me about his diet. An inhabitant of skid row, he drank whatever he could get his hands on and tried to stay drunk all the time. Now and then he consumed a bottle of sweet red wine, but mostly he stuck to whiskey or rum. He couldn't recall having eaten a balanced meal in years.

The task of returning Walter's blood to normal took several weeks. His needs were so great that we gave him injections of iron and vitamins, but we aimed much of our therapy at showing him how to build his blood by eating right.

The Importance of Eating to Build the Blood in Every Way

In addition to iron, the body needs the following vitamins to build rich red blood:

- *Folic acid.* To put plenty of folic acid into your diet, eat green, leafy vegetables every day. However, cooking can remove the folic acid from vegetables. You can get around this by eating the vegetables raw or by saving and using the broth when you cook vegetables. Other excellent sources of folic acid are fruits, grains, nuts, milk, cheese, eggs and liver.

- *Vitamin B₁₂.* The richest source of B_{12} is liver. However, ample supplies of this vitamin are present in most meats and in milk, eggs and cheese.

- *Vitamin C.* Vitamin C helps you to absorb iron from your diet and also works to build up your red blood cells and blood vessels. Citrus fruits are rich in vitamin C, and so are many vegetables—especially tomatoes, red peppers and greens.

How Mary S. Solved Her Iron-Deficiency the Effortless Way

Mary S., 40, visited her doctor because of heavy menstrual bleeding. She also gave a history of undue tiredness, and the physician soon discovered why. Mary had severe iron-deficiency anemia. The mother of three, she had enjoyed good health until about a year before her check-up. That was when the heavy bleeding had begun, and it had been getting steadily worse each month. Mary's diet was excellent. She ate plenty of iron, but she had been losing so much blood that her body was unable to absorb iron quickly enough to keep her from becoming anemic.

Mary's gynecologist performed an operation known as a D & C—a scraping out of the inner lining of the uterus (womb). This corrected the excessive menstrual bleeding. The physician also placed Mary on iron pills, and within a few months her blood count had returned to normal.

Getting at the Bottom of Blood Loss

Normally, red blood cells live in the body for about four
months. Then the cells die and are removed from the circulation.
The iron from the broken-down blood cells is saved by the body
for use in making new red blood cells. In this way, you use body
iron over and over. Bleeding, on the other hand, removes iron
from the body. It is lost—gone forever. This is why it is so important to check for any sources of blood loss if you develop iron-
deficiency anemia. The anemia could be a symptom of heavy
menstrual bleeding, chronic nosebleeds, blood loss from the
urinary tract, or even bleeding from a cancer in the bowel. These
are things your doctor can check for, and to avoid the possibility
of overlooking them *you should never begin to treat your own
anemia without first having a medical check-up!* (A medical check-
up is not necessary, however, if you are not anemic and just wish
to build rich red blood for better health. If you think you might be
anemic, the doctor can do a blood test that will tell for sure.)

The problem that can develop when you take iron tablets to
correct an iron-deficiency anemia, and do not first check with your
physician, is illustrated by the case of

The Man Who Won the Battle but Lost the War

Hector R. was 80 years old and independent. You don't get to
be 80 without learning a few things, and Hector felt that he had
learned a lot about doctoring himself. That is why when he began
to feel sluggish and tired all the time he diagnosed iron-deficiency
anemia, purchased some iron tablets and began taking them. Sure
enough, the tablets helped. Within a few weeks Hector felt better.
But he had not seen the end of his problem. Four months after he
began to take the iron tablets he developed such bad constipation
that he went to the doctor for help. The physician quickly saw the
problem. Hector had cancer of the large intestine, and the cancer
had completely obstructed the intestinal tract. During a four-hour
operation the surgeon relieved the obstruction, but he couldn't
remove all of the cancer. It had spread to the liver.

Hector's anemia had come from bleeding into the intestine,
and by doctoring it with iron tablets he had given the cancer an ad-

ditional four months to grow. The cancer might have been curable if Hector had gone to the doctor at the onset of his anemia. By treating himself with iron tablets, the patient won the battle but lost the war. To repeat the lesson, *if you suspect you are anemic, visit your physician for a check-up.* Anemia is not a disease in and of itself. It is a sign that something is wrong with your health.

Some Things to Watch for

Iron-deficiency anemia is a signal that points to a poor diet or to bleeding. Some possible sources of bleeding that you should watch for and report to your physician are:

1. *Heavy menstrual bleeding.* This is quite common during menopause (ages 45-50). The heavy bleeding can occur between periods or be reflected as an increase in the rate and duration of bleeding each month. The treatment rarely requires anything more difficult than the relatively minor operation known as a D & C.

2. *Bleeding from the rectum.* Bleeding hemorrhoids usually produce bright red blood that appears on the toilet paper or on top of the stool in the commode. Bleeding that comes from somewhere in the intestinal tract has a different appearance. The blood has usually been partially digested and looks black or tarry, or like wine-colored jelly. A bleeding ulcer, a cancer of the bowel and many other conditions can cause bleeding from the rectum.

3. *Nosebleed.* This obvious form of bleeding can be overlooked by an independent-minded person who is determined not to be sick or let the nosebleed interfere with his activities. Nosebleeds in an adult can be serious, and the person suffering nosebleeds should be checked by a physician.

4. *Blood in the urine.* A bladder or kidney infection is the most common cause of blood in the urine. Rarely is the bleeding sufficient to cause iron-deficiency anemia, but it can be. It's a good idea to have the problem investigated by a doctor.

When Taking Iron Tablets Can Be Helpful

Under a doctor's direction, taking iron tablets can be helpful. Women lose about twice as much iron each month as men, and childbirth adds greatly to the iron depletion. Some women in the childbearing years get by much better if they take iron tablets. Strict vegetarians have to take iron tablets to get enough iron, and some persons prefer to take iron instead of eating the foods that contain it. You can buy iron without a prescription. Here are some things to remember about buying this medicine:

- *Ferrous sulfate tablets are the best.* They provide the most iron, and they provide it in a form that is easy for the intestine to absorb.

- *Take the medicine after a meal.* Taking the iron at the end of a meal will help cut down on symptoms such as nausea or upset stomach that might develop otherwise. Most people can get by with taking only two or, at the most, three iron tablets a day.

- *The iron tablets will turn the stool black.* Sometimes it can be difficult to tell whether a very black stool color is due to intestinal bleeding or to iron therapy. However, bleeding generally causes soft, tarry stools, while with iron therapy the stools keep their firmness and tend to have a greenish-black color.

- *Choose a safe place to store the iron tablets.* Iron tablets can be extremely poisonous to youngsters. Keep iron and all other medicines in a locked cabinet out of the reach of children.

Avoiding Blood-Damaging Chemicals

We live in an age of chemistry. Chemicals get into our food as it is grown, and we use chemicals in the processing of food. We put elements such as flouride into our drinking water, and we take chemicals in the form of drugs to have better health. The thing to remember is that drugs are chemicals and that some of them can be harmful. Certain chemicals, in fact, can damage the blood. Let me give as an example the case of

The Woman Who Learned the Hard Way
That Drugs Can Be Bad as Well as Good

Shirley, a 39-year-old black woman, was a telephone operator. One day she noticed that it burned when she passed urine, yet she still had the urge to pass urine every few minutes. A physician diagnosed a bladder infection and prescribed a sulfa drug. A few days later Shirley's burning and frequency of urination were gone, but she had developed a high fever, chills and back pain. Her blood count dropped quite suddenly, and she was admitted to the hospital.

Her doctor realized too late that Shirley was among the 10 or 15% of black people who are susceptible to a type of anemia that can develop suddenly when they are given certain drugs, including sulfa. Shirley recovered, but not until she had received several blood transfusions and had been in the hospital for two weeks.

The condition that led to her problem is known as *G-6-PD deficiency*, and Shirley and others who have this susceptibility to developing anemia should avoid taking:

- *Antimalarial drugs such as primaquine or quinine*
- *Sulfa drugs such as sulfanilamide or sulfisoxazole*
- *Nitrofurantoin*
- *Aspirin in high doses*

Some chemicals are capable of causing the blood count to drop even when the person does not have an inherited trait such as G-6-PD deficiency. Chloramphenicol, an antibiotic, suppresses the blood-forming tissues of almost everyone who takes it. And on rare occasions this antibiotic produces a very serious and often fatal condition known as aplastic anemia. Other drugs that can damage your blood cells are phenylbutazone, propylthiouracil, mephenytoin, methyldopa, aminopyrine, gold salts and anticancer drugs. You can use two rules to minimize your risk of taking one of these potentially hazardous drugs:

Rule One: Do not take any medicine unless you have a specific need for it.

Rule Two: Choose a physician who understands the potential harmfulness of drugs.

In the opinion of your doctor, the condition for which he is treating you may warrant the use of a potentially harmful drug. On the other hand, a doctor who is worth your trust won't mind you asking about the potential harmfulness of any drug. One final note: Never, under any circumstances, take medicines from someone else's prescription. It was once my sad experience to care for a woman who died from drug-induced anemia. She developed the anemia and low white blood cell count from taking aminopyrine to relieve a mild fever. The drug had been prescribed for her husband, not her. This unfortunate woman would have suffered less if she had taken a bottle of arsenic.

How Adelle Turned a Simple Treatment into a Blood-Building Process

Adelle W., a 56-year-old editor for a textbook publishing firm, stayed too busy to devote much time to her health. During the day she worked, evenings she liked to read, and on weekends she did some writing of her own. Her only medical problem was sinusitis, and she neglected it. She was surprised to learn while offering to donate a unit of blood to the blood bank, that she was mildly anemic.

She rarely visited a doctor, but she decided to have the anemia investigated. The physician could find no obvious cause for the problem and referred her to a blood specialist. I was working with the specialist at the time and was myself puzzled by the editor's anemia.

"What about the sinusitis?" the specialist asked.

I admitted that it showed up on her x-rays and that she tended to neglect it.

"Well, a chronic infection like this can cause anemia. We don't understand how it does so, but the infection suppresses formation of blood cells. I'll bet if we can get her sinusitis cleared up we can cure Adelle's anemia."

The blood specialist was right. It took some time, and the help of an allergist and an ear, nose, and throat specialist, but at a return visit a year later, Adelle's blood count was near normal. "I thought my sinusitis was just something I had to live with," she said. "Now I have it under control, and my head feels better and I feel stronger because my blood count's normal."

Taking Advantage of the Fact That
Clearing Up Disease in One Part of Your Body
Can Help the Rest of You

If you suffer from a smoldering infection somewhere in your body, removing this infection will allow your blood count to build back to normal. Among the infections that can cause anemia are:

- Lung infections
- Sinusitis
- Kidney and bladder infections
- Sores or ulcers

It makes sense to bring these infections under control! Your doctor is the best person to prescribe appropriate therapy.

The Neglected Ingredient You
Can Use to Build Rich Red Blood

People who live at high altitudes, such as in Denver, Colorado, tend to have richer, redder blood than persons living at sea level, such as in New Orleans or Miami. The reason is that the air is thinner in Denver, and the local citizens respond by building up a correspondingly greater blood count. You don't have to move to Denver, however, to enrich your blood. You can take advantage of the same mechanism by using a neglected ingredient to boost your blood count. This neglected ingredient is . . . EXERCISE!

A Trick You Can Learn from the Athletes

The 1968 Olympic Games were held in Mexico City. Mexico City is built on a plateau 7,440 feet above sea level—almost half a mile higher than Denver. Unaware that the high altitude would affect their performance, some athletes trained at sea level until just before the Games. They did poorly, and some of the runners fainted just after a race or during it. These persons had not given themselves time to develop the extra number of red blood cells they needed to compete at high altitudes. The winning athletes almost invariably turned out to be the ones who had trained for several months in Mexico City before the games or who had found a high-altitude training spot in their own country. Doing so made sense in winning or doing well in a race, and you can use the same technique to have richer, redder blood.

If you were to move from Miami to Denver, for example, your blood would grow richer to make up for the thinness of the air. You can benefit from the same effect without moving anywhere, and you can enrich your blood even if you already live in the mile-high city. *You do it by exercising regularly.* Exercise puts your red blood cells to work. It stimulates them in much the same way as does living at a high altitude. The result of regular exercise is a strengthening of your blood and a toning up of your body. In other words, you benefit from exercise in the same way that any fine machine benefits from being kept in tune.

Chapters 4, 5 and 6 give details on developing a regular, personal exercise program. In these chapters, too, you can learn that exercising helps fight fatigue and boost the vitality of your heart and vessels. Eating foods that build the blood can also build the health of other parts of your body. In other words, doing one thing to have better health gives back several dividends in return. What this can mean is that you'll stay healthy and young and enjoy the longevity that you deserve.

2

Deriving Energy from the Things That Used to Make You Tired

Tiredness can be a symptom of many things. Among these are anemia, a low-grade infection, thyroid disease, heart failure and liver disease. The first step in correcting the symptom is a medical checkup; if your physician can find no evidence of disease, then it may be that a change in your life style is the right prescription!

The four ways you can derive energy from the things that used to make you tired are:

1. *Add new activities to your life.*
2. *Draw energy from a regular exercise program.*
3. *Lose weight if you are overweight.*
4. *Relax and get the rest you need.*

Mae's Discovery of a Quick Way to Have Energy in Abundance

Mae, a 50-year-old housewife, thought she had cancer. In the mornings, when she should have been at her freshest, she felt tired. The fatigue lasted through the day, and she was often too tired to fix dinner for her husband. Mae sighed deeply as she told me, "I just feel tired."

A clinical examination and laboratory tests showed that Mae did not have cancer. Her heart, lungs and breasts were in good health, and her figure was trim and attractive. She seemed disappointed to hear these results and told me so. "Something just has to be wrong with me, doctor. Else why would I feel this way?" She went on to explain that the youngest of her four children, a daughter, had just graduated from college, gotten married and moved to another state. Her other children were busy with their own lives, and her husband's work seemed to be taking more and more of his time. In short, her life had slowed down and left her with an empty feeling. The years of relaxation she had looked forward to for so long were not going to be happy years, she had decided, and she had reached the point of dreading each day.

Mae's tiredness was a symptom of a mild depression, and what she needed more than medicine was *something to do*. Happily, I knew of the crying need for volunteers at a nearby state school for the mentally retarded. Mae was skeptical about working there, but went anyway. She took to it instantly. It gave her something to do each day, a reason for being, and she began to plan her other activities around her work at the school. Last time I saw her, Mae was the Director of Volunteer Services at the school. She had done nothing less than start a new career at the age of fifty. She told me she was happier than she had ever been! Fatigue was something she could barely remember.

Taking Advantage of Three Quick Sources of Energy

Nothing is better for you than change. Boredom breeds discontent, and fatigue and boredom go hand in hand. Change, the simple act of doing something different, can bring back the freshness and vigor you used to feel! Here are three ways to derive energy by changing something in your life:

1. *Take a trip.* Go somewhere! And not only that, go somewhere you haven't been before! Just the notion of getting away is often enough to start new energy flowing through your body. In fact, by beginning to plan the trip you can start your enjoyment immediately. Visit the place you have always dreamed of visiting, and if necessary, go alone! You'll meet new people, get a new look at yourself, bring new experiences into your life. Taking a trip is one of the quickest ways to rid yourself of fatigue and boredom.

2. *Take a new job.* Fatigue can accompany a dread of going to work or facing the day's activities. So change! Find

something else to do. We human beings sometimes tend to take ourselves too seriously; we claim we can't do anything differently, because who would do what we have been doing? In fact, things can and will go on without you, and you may be surprised at how well! By the same token, getting a new hold on your life will make you a more effective individual. I know of an electrical engineer who gave up the rat race and is now happily selling bicycles, an attorney who gave up a lucrative law practice to become a sportswriter, and a school teacher who quit the classroom to become a nature photographer. Many, many women have given up full-time housework to take a job and are happy they have done so. The point is this: If you are unhappy, changing what you do can make a world of difference by bringing some bounce back into your life.

3. *Find a new friend.* Promise yourself that within the next few days you are going to make a new friend and that the two of you will do something together. Like to read? Find someone who wants to accompany you to the library. Or you can bowl together or sew together or visit the sick or shop or go for a drive or eat lunch or take a walk together. Or fall in love, for that matter. The important thing is that you bring a new person into your life. It will give you energy, and it will give you a reason for being. And don't worry if you consider yourself shy. Make the initial effort, and the other person will surprise you by meeting you more than half way.

How to Have Power in Reserve

Scheduling new activities is bound to give you energy, and one particular form of activity, exercise, can give you power in reserve. Before I began exercising regularly I was extremely tired at the end of the day, even though my job was not taxing—I taught physiology classes at a large university. A man who taught in the same department felt just the opposite from me. He never got tired. One day he surprised me by asking if I wanted to accompany him on a jogging session during lunch.

"Now wait a minute,"I said, "you have all this energy, and on top of that you jog? And during the lunch hour? How do you make it through the rest of the day?"

"The secret is that I couldn't make it if I *didn't* exercise! Far from making me tired, it gives me energy. If I couldn't exercise every day, I don't know how I'd make it."

Since then, I have learned that he was right. In a nutshell, what exercise does is pep you up and give you more energy than you need for your ordinary activities. Let me use the common foot race as an example. If you were on the track team and your specialty was the mile run, your coach would not have you train to run only one mile. Why not? Because to do your best in a one-mile race, you have to train at running two or three miles. Then, because your body is so well-trained, you can run the mile race with ease (and speed). Your daily activities represent the race you run every day. Exercise, by conditioning your body to do more than your ordinary activities, makes it easier for you to accomplish your day's work. Begin exercising, and you'll feel new power flowing through your veins; you'll have a new spring in your step; you'll bubble with energy. To repeat, you'll feel this way because exercise trains your body to do more than you would ordinarily ask of it.

Learning to Draw Power from Natural Sources

But how can you exercise if you're tired? It's true, when you feel tired you don't want to exercise. On the other hand, the very time you need to exercise is when your feet feel like lead weights and there is no reason for them to feel this way. If you are in good health and getting enough rest, a feeling of sluggishness during the day is a call for activity. Only a few minutes into your exercise session you'll feel better. Movement stimulates your circulation and invigorates your nerves! You think more clearly. You feel refreshed. The human body was built to move about, to bend and twist and walk and stretch, and it feels better when it is used. The heart and circulation, the joints, the muscles, the feet, the arms, the brain—every part of the body benefits from movement. The power you gain from exercising will enter your body like a new surge of energy. People the world over are discovering the invigorating, youth-giving effects of exercise.

The Man Who Discovered That Exercise
Is Better Than Any Drug

John W., a 46-year-old executive who worked in a state office building, came to me for treatment of high blood pressure. John was one of the most frustrated persons I have ever met. His high blood pressure was not his only problem. He couldn't get along with his boss. Their work involved supervising about 20 employees who handled complaints from motorists who felt they had been treated unfairly by highway patrol officers, park rangers or other agents whose jobs were to enforce state laws. John's boss was more a hindrance than a help in the effort to keep the office running smoothly. The boss came to work late, was sloppy in his personal habits, and drank. And if something went wrong, he was quick to blame it on my patient.

"Sometimes I feel like I'm going to explode," my patient said, "and other times I get up in the morning and feel so dead tired I don't think I can go to work."

I sympathized with the patient and his problem and made a suggestion. "I've noticed they're building a new highway behind the building where you work. Why don't you take some exercise clothes to work with you and then, right after you get off work, put them on and get out on that clear stretch of land? You've told me how frustrated you usually feel at the end of the day. Well, get out there and walk and jog a little, and let yourself unlimber. You can do it while the other people are fighting the traffic to get home. You'll lose some weight, your exercising will help keep your blood pressure down, and most of all you're going to get over that feeling of tiredness you have each morning."

He followed my suggestion, and it worked. "Doctor, that exercising is better than any drug you could take for pep up. I get out there and smell the fresh air and unlimber my muscles, and I can just feel the problems draining away. I love my work, and I believe exercise is the best way I've ever found of coping with the stress in a healthy way."

The story has a happy ending. The troublesome boss showed up drunk on the job one time too many. His inebriation was discovered by *his* boss, and he was forced to take early retirement. My patient became the new boss, and he still derives energy (and keeps his blood pressure down) by continuing a regular exercise program.

Three Ways to Make Pepping Up a Habit

The best form of exercise for you will depend on your particular likes and dislikes; the availability of parks, swimming pools and gyms; and the amount of time you can devote to an exercise program. Walking is the exercise I will stress most in this book, because it is so universally available and inexpensive. But for any exercise to pep you up, you need to make it a habit. This means doing it every day, planning it in your schedule. Here are three ways to do this:

1. *Begin the day with an exercise session.* Start each day with a nice, brisk walk right in your neighborhood. Doing so will give you more energy for the day's activities. Many people enjoy this early morning habit, but if you aren't one of them you can . . .

2. *Take a walk in the evening.* John W. enjoyed doing his exercise right after work, while his fellow workers were fighting the traffic home. This method might work for you, but if you are the sort who would rather go straight home, plan your walk for right after dinner. Besides pepping you up, a walk after the evening meal will help you digest your food.

3. *Exercise twice as much on weekends.* Even if you are retired you probably have more free time on weekends than during the week. Saturdays and Sundays are the times to walk in earnest, to get out of doors and enjoy life. Maybe you can combine the weekend exercise with another activity, such as birdwatching. Get some binoculars and a guide book and see how many different species you can identify (there are 15,000 species of birds in the world).

The Woman Who Reshaped Her Life by Reshaping Her Body

Norma A., 52, was overweight, unhappy and tired. It was difficult for me to tell whether she was unhappy because she was overweight, or overweight because she was unhappy. The thing that bothered Norma most, however, was her fatigue. When she felt tired she stopped her activities and thus tended to gain more weight. One of her problems was that she was convinced that energy comes from what you eat rather than from what you do.

"Surely you must know that the extra 60 pounds you're carrying around add to your fatigue," I told her. "How'd you like to go around all day with a fully loaded camping pack on your back? That's what you're doing."

"Yes, but I eat a healthy breakfast. That's suppose to give me energy."

"Does it?"

She shook her head.

"The reason you don't have any energy," I told Norma, "is that the kind of energy that makes you want to do things doesn't come from what you eat. *It comes from the things you do every day and from having a healthy body weight.*" We discussed weight loss, exercise and the natural ways to draw power from natural sources. I was able to help my patient understand that the way to overcome fatigue is to have power in reserve, power that comes from having a trim, well-exercised body. Norma had never been able to lose weight on her own, but with the help of Weight Watchers she was able to lose 30 pounds, and she has continued on the Weight Watchers program. I don't see her as a patient any more, but recently I did run into her in a shopping mall. She was more excited than I had ever seen her.

"I'm shopping for a size 14 dress, and if I keep losing I'll buy one that's even smaller. And doctor, you were so right! I have more energy just from losing 30 pounds than I've had since high school, and that was over 30 years ago! The nicest thing is that the better I feel the more I want to do, and the more I do the quicker I can lose weight. And that makes me feel better and helps me with my diet. It's wonderful!"

Accomplishing Many Things by Doing One

Losing weight if you are obese can do more than just provide you with a new surge of energy. It can lower your blood pressure, boost the vitality of your heart and vessels, and keep you from having diabetes, varicose veins and swelling of the feet and ankles. Losing weight and keeping it off is such an important subject that Chapter 6 is devoted to it.

Ed S.'s Remedy for Insomnia and Fatigue

Ed slept all right some of the time, but at other times he had trouble falling off. He was a 45-year-old salesman, and he felt that if he didn't get enough sleep he'd face the day tired and unable to be at his peak. So Ed began taking sleeping pills. At first he got some of the ones you see advertised on TV, but they didn't work very well. Ed borrowed some prescription sleeping pills from a friend and found that they worked much better—for a week or two. Then, one sleeping pill didn't do the trick any more. After taking the pill Ed would lie down and toss and turn uncomfortably, unable to get to sleep. Why not try two sleeping pills? He did. Two pills put Ed to sleep, but then instead of feeling fresh the next morning he felt groggy and hungover from the medicine. It was at this point that Ed had the good sense to visit his physician.

"It's a good thing you came in, Ed," the doctor told him, "because you were on the road to being addicted to those sleeping pills. People get started taking them and don't know how to stop. There are two things you need to remember about getting to sleep. In the first place, it's a natural thing, and it will come to you if you'll wait for it. And in the second place, sleeping pills probably interfere with sleep more than they help it."

Ed S. stopped taking pills to get to sleep, and his sales picked up immediately. Not only did he feel better without the morning hangover of the pills, the natural sleep he began to enjoy proved to be far more refreshing than drugged sleep.

Why the Natural Way Is the Best Way

Your body and your mind need rest each night, and sleep provides this. However, many people who take sleeping pills actually get up the next morning and feel as if they haven't rested. The reason for this is that sleep brought on by drugs is not as refreshing as natural sleep!

Sleep consists of regular cycles and rhythms. Far from "sleeping like a log," you sleep at changing levels of unconsciousness. Dreams, for example, occur during the lightest stage of sleep and can be considered a natural way that the mind "exercises" by resorting to fantasy and adventure that you might not experience during your waking hours. Drugged sleep is unhealthy sleep, for drugs interfere with dreaming and with the normal sleep cycles that are necessary for you to get the rest you need. One consequence of drugged sleep is that the person who relies on sleeping pills soon stops dreaming—or experiences nightmares as the effects of the drug wear off.

The natural way to rest and sleep is the best way. Even some of the over-the-counter sleeping aids that are advertised on television can be very dangerous if you take too many of them. This was brought home to me by the case of

The Girl Who Took Too Many

She did it to commit suicide, and she succeeded. But she didn't take a barbiturate or another of the potent prescription sleeping pills. She took about 18 capsules of a commonly advertised sleeping aid that is available without a prescription. The drug contained a chemical that damaged her brain's temperature control center. Her body temperature soared to 110°, and the high temperature led to kidney failure. The patient died less than a week after taking the overdose of "mild" sleeping aids.

This unfortunate event underscores the point that too much of any medicine can be dangerous and that even the so-called "safe" sleeping aids can be very harmful.

How to Fill Your Life with the Energy That Comes from Natural Sleep

You can get the sleep you need, and you can get it naturally! Here are five ways to do so:

#1. MAKE SLEEP A HABIT.

Build good sleeping habits. This means going to bed at about the same time every night, whether or not you feel sleepy. Even if you don't drop right off, let your mind relax. Many people who consider themselves insomniacs actually sleep more than they believe they do. We have all had the feeling of thinking we were awake only to realize when someone says something or switches on a light that we were actually dozing. In a dark room with your body comfortable on the bed, you'll sleep. Remember that sleep operates on a supply and demand basis. Failing to go right to sleep one night will probably enable you to drop right off the next. No one ever died from a lack of sleep!

#2. PROVIDE YOURSELF SOME PEACE AND QUIET.

Make your sleeping area as comfortable as possible. If you sleep with a partner and are cramped for space, consider purchasing a king-sized bed. If your partner snores or moves around so much that he or she awakens you during the night, get twin beds—or sleep in a separate room. Some people enjoy going to sleep to the drone of a small fan next to the bed. In the winter the fan may seem unnecessary, but it can help drown out the automatic on-and-off cycling of the central heating fan.

#3. PREPARE YOURSELF TO SLEEP.

Begin calming down before bedtime. Don't watch a hotly contested game or an exciting movie on TV and then expect to fall right to sleep. Try to save family disagreements for the following day—when, most likely, the problem will seem much smaller anyway. Spend the last hour or two before bedtime preparing yourself to sleep. Read a book (not a suspense novel), talk quietly or relax to music. Some radio stations play soothing music late at night, and you may want to purchase a radio that will automatically shut itself off after you go to sleep listening to music.

#4. LEARN TO COUNT SHEEP.

Once in bed, try not to dwell on problems or worries. This isn't always easy, but with practice you can accomplish it. Perhaps you can benefit from forming a mental picture of yourself walking over to a precipice and casting your worries down the side of the cliff and away from you forever—or at least until the next morning! Concentrate on thinking pleasant thoughts.

Begin by trying to remember the most pleasurable thing you've done in the past week or month. Go over it again and again in your mind; dwell on it. Plan to repeat it. *Promise yourself that you will repeat it!* Or, try thinking of an open field with grass swaying lazily in a gentle breeze, or a lone kite high and magnificent in a blue sky, a kite that starts to fall and fall and fall . . . . Or pretend your body is a sack of potatoes: Suddenly someone splits the bottom of the sack, and the potatoes begin to tumble out. Feel yourself relaxing? You get the idea.

#5. AVOID STIMULANTS.

If you have trouble sleeping, don't have coffee or tea in the evenings. In fact, it's best not to eat anything at all for at least two hours before retiring.

Pills you took earlier in the day can interfere with sleep. Pep-up pills (speed) stimulate the nervous system. Sometimes these pills are prescribed to help someone lose weight, but they can keep the person from getting to sleep at night. The best way to prevent this is not to take stimulant drugs of any kind. Should your doctor put you on a weight-reducing drug, you'll need to avoid taking it after four or so in the afternoon. Better yet, don't take drugs to help you lose weight. At best their effect is temporary, and at worst they can elevate your blood pressure, make you constipated, cause you to be nervous—and keep you awake at nights. Besides that, stimulant drugs are habit-forming.

Getting the Rest You Need

How much sleep you should get depends on your body's needs. Eight or nine hours of sleep is average, but as you get older you may need less sleep than you did ten or fifteen years earlier. Here's how to tell if you're getting the rest you need. If it always takes the alarm to drag you out of bed, your rhythms are off. If you're getting the sleep you need, you ought to wake up each morning on your own.

Train yourself to sleep normally, expect to sleep normally, and if you are in harmony with yourself and your environment you'll look forward to a good night's sleep—every night.

3

How to Have Better Health from What You Eat

You are what you eat! And you can enjoy better health from eating nutritious, strength-giving foods. The diet that is right for you will depend on many things, and my purpose in this chapter is to offer tips on healthy eating for the entire family and to show how individual diets can work to cure or relieve certain medical problems.

What You Eat Does Make a Difference

Food is a big part of our lives. To some persons food is a religious or social tradition, to others it is the reward for a hard day's work, and to almost all of us it represents love and sharing and family life at its happiest. Food should be enjoyed, but eating is too important an activity to let enjoyment be the only guide. You need to know about foods, about the products that can give you good health and those that work against your health. The four food groups are:

1. *Meats*—beef, veal, poultry, fish and liver
2. *Fruits and vegetables*—citrus and other fruits; green vegetables and yellow vegetables
3. *Breads and cereals*—bread made from grain; hot or cold cereals
4. *The milk group*—milk, cheese, yogurt, ice cream and margarine

Ideally, you ought to eat foods from each of these groups every day. However, some of the food groups are more important than others. You can more easily and healthily do without the milk group, for example, than you can do without meats, fruits and vegetables, or breads and cereals. Also, foods within the various groups differ in their quality and in their potential to give you good health. Stop at the meat counter of a supermarket and look over the array of different cuts: steak, roast, veal cutlet, ground round, brisket and tongue. Farther down the counter you'll find pork, poultry, liver and fish. Some of these meats are chock-full of fat and cholesterol—substances capable of causing fatty deposits in your heart and arteries. Other meats are lean and low in fat and cholesterol, and they are thus much better health bargains. Having better health from what you eat begins, then, with knowing what foods to buy and set on the table.

Seven Tips to Save You Money
and Improve Your Health

TIP #1. LEAN MEAT IS HEALTHIER THAN THICK, JUICY STEAKS.

The thicker and juicier the steak, the more fat it contains. The fat content of meat is dangerous for two reasons. Fats give you more than twice as many calories as carbohydrates or proteins, and thus they make you gain weight more easily. The more important reason for choosing lean meat, however, is that by avoiding fatty meats you automatically lower your intake of saturated fats and cholesterol. A high intake of saturated fats and cholesterol is believed to be one of the main causes of coronary artery disease, heart attack, and diseases of the arteries such as stroke and poor circulation.

TIP #2. INEXPENSIVE BREAKFAST FOODS ARE ALSO THE BEST BREAKFAST FOODS.

Sausage, bacon and ham are expensive, and these meats are also the worst things you can eat for breakfast! They are loaded with saturated fats and cholesterol. The eggs that go with sausage, bacon and ham are not too expensive, but eggs are high in fats and can contribute to heart disease. Cereals, toast and juice are much less expensive—and promote your health rather than damaging it! Let me give you an example of what I mean.

How Ed S. Got Each Day
Started the Right Way
with a Healthy Breakfast

Ed S., 55, was a career Air Force noncommissioned officer. I got to know him when he came in for a routine preretirement physical examination. I was surprised at Ed's good health. He looked to be no more than 40 years old, was trim and strong and full of energy.

"What'd you eat for breakfast this morning?" I asked him.

"One slice of toast with jelly and one cup of coffee."

"And that's all?"

"Doctor, about the only time I change it is when I have a biscuit or two instead of the toast, and some mornings I have juice along with the coffee."

I asked Ed to explain why he chose to eat a light rather than a heavy breakfast.

"For one thing, I keep from gaining weight that way. There's no way you can eat three big meals and hold your own unless you do a good workout every day. Actually, I do exercise. I try to walk three miles a day and go by the gym several times a week for a workout. But skipping all those fatty breakfast foods lets me eat more at supper. And to tell the truth, I just feel better on a light breakfast."

I learned something from my patient; in the ten years since I met Ed, I've enjoyed the benefits of eating a light, healthy breakfast. I've discussed with many persons the pros and cons of a light morning meal. The main point I have to make is that

The Energy for Your Day Doesn't Come
from What You Eat for Breakfast

Breakfast doesn't give you energy! If anything, a heavy breakfast can make you feel sluggish. The get-up-and-go feeling all of us want to have each day depends not on what we eat but on how we feel. And that morning boost of energy comes from having good mental and physical health! An invigorating desire to get things done is far more dependent on the tone and rhythm and health of your body than on what foods you eat for breakfast. A regular exercise program, reducing to your ideal weight and keeping your body at peak efficiency are far better "energizers" than eating bacon and eggs for breakfast.

On the other hand, perhaps you enjoy a big breakfast too much to give it up. Or maybe you do hard physical labor and need something in your stomach. Okay. Eat a big breakfast, but make it an energizing meal. Keep the foods light and the portions medium or small. Eat fruit or fruit juice, coffee or tea, and oatmeal, cream of wheat or the cereal of your choice. Enjoy toast or biscuits with the meal. Do keep in mind that children need a relatively larger breakfast than adults. But children do not need to eat sausage, bacon, ham or eggs!

TIP #3. SELECT NATURAL FOODS RATHER THAN PROCESSED ONES.

Processed foods are treated with preservatives and then packaged, bottled or canned so that they won't spoil while sitting on the grocer's shelf. Chemicals are added to processed foods as preservatives or to make the food look pretty. An example is red dye food coloring, used to color cookies, canned fruits, jello, wieners and hundreds of other items. Research in the mid-1970's showed that the dye caused cancer in mice, and the Food and Drug Administration banned its use. But red dye is only one of literally thousands of different chemicals that get into processed foods—and thus into the human body. Among the processed foods to avoid, and the foods to buy instead, are:

Stay away from	Okay
Cold cuts, frankfurters	Peanut butter
Salami, potted meat	Lean veal, low-fat ground beef
Potato chips, corn chips	Wheat germ, whole grain cereal
White bread	Whole wheat or whole rye bread
TV dinners	Fresh fruits, fresh meats, fresh vegetables

TIP #4. PUT FISH AND POULTRY INTO YOUR DIET.

Protein is the main building substance of the body. Your body needs protein to form healthy bones, muscle and skin. Meat is a fine source of protein, but many persons overlook the fact that fish and poultry can supply as much protein as a similar cut of beef—and at a savings of calories and money. A three-ounce serving of haddock fillet, for example, supplies only 150 calories to your diet. Yet it contains about as much protein as three ounces of pork chops or beefsteak. The pork chops give you 375 calories, and the beefsteak provides 430—almost three times as many calories as in the cut of fish. Chicken and other poultry are also low in calories and yet rich in protein.

Beans and rice are two excellent sources of protein. In fact, a meatless meal can be built around beans and rice, and one or two such meals a week not only won't hurt you, it will give you better health than eating roast, steak or other rich meats. Putting fish and poultry into your diet protects your heart, may help you to lose weight, and can have added benefits for certain individuals.

Raymond's Discovery of a Diet That
Prevented His Attacks of Joint Pain

Raymond was 60 years old, obese, and howling with pain. They brought him to the emergency room in an ambulance, because the pain in his big toe was so bad he couldn't walk. The previous night he had gone to a banquet, and he woke up with the pain in his toe next morning. All day it kept getting worse, but Raymond put off seeing a doctor; he was a politician and wanted to attend another banquet that night. He didn't make it. His toe swelled to three times its normal size, and Raymond came to the hospital.

I diagnosed the problem as an attack of gout, and Raymond spent a miserable night in the hospital waiting for the medicine I gave him to take effect. The drug was colchicine, and at about the same time that it finally relieved my patient's pain, it also triggered a severe attack of diarrhea. I explained to Raymond that colchicine almost always caused diarrhea, that loose stools were a troublesome side effect of the medicine.

"What I want to know," the politician asked me, "is how I can keep from getting the gout again? I don't want to have that pain any more, and I don't want to go through the side effects of taking that medicine."

I explained that there was no cure for gout and that Raymond could take a pill that would lessen his risk of having another attack. I also pointed out something else: "You can do two other things to reduce your risk of having another attack of gout. One is to lose weight, and the other is to go on a diet. Those two drinks before dinner and the one or two afterwards have to go. That banquet food is too rich for you, especially the meats and gravies. You'll need to stay away from rich steak and roast and to avoid things like liver, kidney, sweetbreads and anchovies."

A few weeks later I saw Raymond again. For an attack of gout. Medicine relieved his pain, but once again caused diarrhea. "Doctor, I didn't stay on that diet," the patient confessed. "I just go to too many different things to watch what I eat. I have to worry constantly about keeping the voters happy."

I suggested Raymond do something I had read that John F. Kennedy used to do. That is, eat *before* a banquet or dinner and then talk or visit during the meal itself. But I cautioned my patient to build his meals around chicken and certain types of fish rather than around the rich foods he obviously preferred. Fortunately, Raymond followed my suggestion. We moved to a different city, and I eventually lost track of him, but I do know that he had no further attacks of gout during the six months I was able to follow him.

TIP #5. FRUITS MAKE A BETTER DESSERT THAN PASTRIES.

Pies, puddings, cookies and cake are fun to eat, but these dessert items are expensive and loaded with fats. Fats contain over twice as many calories as the same weight of carbohydrates. Fruits are carbohydrates, and they can make a delicious dessert that is much less costly than bakery items. Serve fresh fruits mixed with fruit cocktail or sprinkled with diced coconut and wheat germ.

TIP #6. EMPHASIZE A DRINK THAT IS HEALTHIER THAN CARBONATED BEVERAGES.

The drink is water! Few people will dispute that when you are really thirsty, nothing tastes as good as water. But we tend to overlook water in planning meals. A cold glass of water is an excellent drink, especially during the warm spring and summer months. Drinking one or two soft drinks a day is not an unhealthy habit, but water is less expensive and saves you the 150 calories in each can or bottle of regular soda.

TIP #7. SWITCH TO LOW-FAT MILK.

Milk is one of our most dearly loved foods. However, most Americans drink more of it than they actually need, and certain kinds of milk can be unhealthy. These are buttermilk, cream and whole milk. If you drink milk, make it low-fat or skim milk. Low-fat milk is less expensive than regular milk, and it is better for you. The reason for this will be discussed in more detail in Chapter 5.

Taking Advantage of Martha's "Magic" Cure for Diabetes

Martha Y. was a 50-year-old woman I treated during my postgraduate training in internal medicine. She was overweight and a diabetic. She had given birth to three children and had gained weight with each pregnancy—weight she never lost. At age 35, for example, she was admitted to the hospital because of a kidney infection, and doctors discovered glucose in her urine. She was found to have diabetes. At that time Martha weighed 215 pounds, and she had continued to gain weight. Her chart was thick. It told of frequent kidney infections, of diabetic complications, of insulin reactions, of diets she was given but did not follow.

Young and enthusiastic, I took a special interest in trying to get Martha to lose weight. I failed. She seemed to prefer taking insulin for her diabetes, even after I explained time and again that if she would lose weight, chances were that her diabetes would come under control by itself—without the need for insulin injections or other medicine.

I lost track of Martha and then rediscovered her. She came into the hospital one day about two and a half years after I had last seen her, but I didn't recognize my former patient. She wasn't sick, she was there with one of her children.

"What's the matter, Dr. Deaton?" this strange-appearing woman said, "don't you remember me?" I could not, until she refreshed my memory.

"I used to have diabetes, and you and I would fight about my weight every time you saw me in diabetic clinic. Well, I finally got to thinking about what you said and made up my mind to follow your advice. I've lost a hundred and ten pounds and haven't needed a shot of insulin in eight months. They discharged me from diabetic clinic."

That was Martha—a new woman and no longer a diabetic. Even though in regaining her health she had followed my advice (and that of many other doctors), her case was astonishing to me. It was as if everything I had told her was theoretical—until she proved the truth of my "theory" by actually losing weight and getting over her diabetes. It was an amazing fact.

Diseases That Eating Right Can Prevent or "Cure"

Just as what you eat can make a difference to your health, so can *how much* you eat. Martha had grown up in a family of heavy eaters, and food was abundant in the home she and her husband provided for their children. One reason Martha let herself get fat was her tendency to eat to relieve a headache or an upset stomach or a case of the blues. It is true that eating right can give you better health; at the same time, obesity is a danger signal that means you have not been eating right! Excess weight is the most preventable of all diseases, and Chapter 6 is devoted to showing you how to lose weight and keep it off. Other conditions that you can control or even "cure" by how you handle yourself at the dinner table include:

- Diabetes
- Heart disease
- High blood pressure
- Swelling of the legs
- Osteoarthritis
- Varicose veins
- Chronic kidney failure
- Chronic liver failure
- Food allergies

I used the word "cure" with a note of caution, which is why I put it in quotation marks. The signs of Martha's diabetes, for example, went away when she lost one hundred pounds. Her urine no longer contained sugar, her blood level of sugar became normal, and she no longer had to give herself injections of insulin. Yet whether her diabetes was "cured" was a matter of opinion. Should she regain the weight she lost, the diabetes would undoubtedly return. What I am saying is this: Reducing to your ideal weight and eating the right foods can help any of the conditions listed above. But whether the condition is "cured" or not depends on whether you continue the healthy eating and keep your body weight at an ideal level. Dietary treatment of most of these conditions will be discussed in other parts of this book. This chapter will take up food allergies and the way to prevent the symptoms of these allergic reactions.

Food Allergies and How to Prevent Them

Food allergies are more common than most people realize. In fact, if you are bothered by nasal congestion, cough, wheezing, chest and throat mucus, skin rash, hives, stomachache or diarrhea, the problem could be a food allergy. You ought to check with a doctor before making a self-diagnosis, but if you do have this problem, elimination of the offending food from your diet is the treatment.

Rosalind's Discovery of How to Prevent Skin Rash

Rosalind, a 32-year-old secretary, had been bothered with hay fever for years. She visited an allergist and took shots to control her sensitivity to ragweed and certain pollens, but she continued to have another problem, a troublesome skin rash on her arms and chest. Finally her doctor put her on an elimination diet, and when Rosalind stopped eating corn and substances made from corn, her rash disappeared.

How Thurmond Overcame His Attacks of Diarrhea

Thurmond, an 18-year-old college premedical student, suffered from diarrhea. He had been investigated by many physicians, but the cause of the diarrhea had never been found. Thurmond came up to discuss his problem after a physiology class I taught, and I suggested that he might have a condition known as *lactase deficiency.* Milk contains a sugar, lactose, and a person's intestine normally contains an enzyme, lactase, that helps to break milk sugar down so that it can be absorbed for use by the body. People who are deficient in lactase (the condition is inherited) develop stomachache and diarrhea when they drink milk or eat milk products. The condition resembles a milk allergy.

It was interesting to me that on his own Thurmond had come to realize that milk seemed to cause his diarrhea. He did not drink milk, but he sometimes ate ice cream or cheese. He had no further trouble with diarrhea after eliminating all milk-containing foods from his diet.

Let Your Symptoms Be Your Guide

The way to find out if you have a food allergy is to go on an elimination diet. List your symptoms on a piece of paper and make a daily note of their presence or absence while you are on the elimination diet. Usually, you will need to eliminate only one food group at a time. The food groups in the diet are listed in order of their frequency in causing food allergies. If you suspect you are allergic to only one food given in the list, eliminate it from your diet for two weeks and see if your symptoms disappear. If you suspect an allergy to more than one food group, remove each of the suspicious foods for two weeks.

Assuming your symptoms are relieved, return individual foods to your diet one at a time, three days apart. When symptoms recur after you've restarted a certain food, you know to eliminate that food from your diet completely. Bear in mind that food allergies are permanent; avoiding the causative food is the only way to prevent the symptoms.

The Elimination Diet (see directions given above)

1. Milk. Any form of milk, including milk products such as ice cream, sherbert and frozen dairy products. Cheese, scrambled eggs, mashed potatoes, cakes, puddings, cookies, doughnuts and other things made with or containing milk. Most breads, biscuits, muffins, waffles and pancakes. Butter and most oleomargarines. (Mazola oleo is milk-free.)

2. *Chocolate and cola drinks.*

3. *Corn.* Corn syrup, such as candies, cookies, some breads, buns, canned fruit, jelly, chewing gum, peanut butter, wieners, sausage, lunch meat, and ice cream. Corn meal, such as baked goods and fish sticks. Corn starch, such as soups, gravies, powdered sugar, corn curls, popcorn, hominy or grits, corn, bourbon, beer, corn flour or corn oil. Baked goods, canned goods and ice cream usually contain corn, but may not say so on the label.

4. *Egg.* Baked goods (unless made without eggs), pancakes, waffles, noodles, mayonnaise, meat loaf, breaded foods, meringue, custard, French toast and icing.

5. *Pea family.* Beans, peas, peanuts, peanut butter, soybean, chili and honey.

6. *Citrus fruits.* Oranges, lemons, limes, tangerines, grapefruits—and their juices.

7. *Tomato.* Tomato juice or paste, chili, catsup, soups and stews.

8. *Wheats and grains.* Oats, barley, rice, rye and anything made with wheat, such as cereals, breads, baked goods, flour, crackers, cakes, doughnuts, cookies, waffles, pancakes, pretzels, ice cream cones, pie crust, rolls, buns, macaroni, spaghetti, noodles and gravy.

9. *Cinnamon.* Spiced cakes or meats, cookies, rolls, pies, candies, apple dishes, cinnamon chewing gum, catsup and chili.

10. *Food colors.* Colored drinks (such as Tang or Kool-aid), medicines, soda pop, bubble gum, some wieners, Jello, popsicles, sherbet, frostings and candy.*

This list does not contain *all* possible offending foods. Read the labels if you aren't sure. And once you've identified the foods to avoid, don't fuss about having to give them up. Think about all the things you can still eat—and without the misery you used to have. Also, unless your allergy is very **severe,** you may be able to break your diet now and then. Some **people** can eat a forbidden food once a week and get by with few or no symptoms. This is especially true when the allergy is to egg or milk.

*This elimination diet is based on one in the article, "What to Do about Food Allergies," by Frederic Speer, M.D., *Consultant*, October, 1973, p. 142. *Used with permission of the publishers.*

4

Taking Advantage of the Natural Ways to Control Your Blood Pressure

High blood pressure has been called the "silent killer," because it is possible to have an elevated blood pressure without experiencing symptoms from it. On the other hand, high blood pressure can cause heart disease, stroke, kidney disease and other problems. You have every reason to want to control your blood pressure, and you can take advantage of five natural blood-pressure-lowering measures. If your blood pressure is normal, these measures can keep it that way. The five ways to lower your blood pressure *without drugs* are:

1. *Cut back on your salt intake.*
2. *Begin a program of regular exercise.*
3. *Take the time to handle stress in a healthy manner.*
4. *Stop smoking.*
5. *Reduce to your ideal body weight.*

How Tom Learned to Lower His Blood Pressure without Drugs

Tom, a 60-year-old plumbing contractor, was a hardworking man who had both good habits and bad habits. He worked six days a week to operate his successful business, and he was looking forward to retirement in a few years. Then, tragedy struck. One night while he was watching television, he developed a severe headache. Spots appeared in front of his eyes, and then he blacked out. His wife couldn't wake him. She rushed him to the hospital, where doctors determined that Tom had suffered a stroke. "His blood pressure is extremely high, " the physician said. "We're doing what we can to lower it, and if we can get it down I think your husband has a good chance of making it."

"I just can't understand," Tom's wife said. "He's never been sick."

"Yes, but he's probably carried that high blood pressure around for years. And he is overweight."

Tom woke up the next day, after medication had returned his blood pressure to near normal. His right side was paralyzed, but within a few weeks he had regained the use of his muscles. A month after his stroke, he left the hospital.

Two weeks later he returned for a check-up, and his doctor was alarmed to find that Tom's blood pressure was once again on the rise. "Are you taking the medicine?" the physician asked.

"I sure am," was the patient's reply.

"Tom," the doctor said, taking a new tact, "while you were in the hospital we kept you on a special diet that restricted your salt intake. Now that you're home you can eat anything you want. Now tell me this. Do you eat a lot of salt? Do you eat salty foods like ham, for example?"

Tom grinned. "I love ham," he said, "but not till I've spread a layer of salt on it to get it to taste right! Salt's a habit with me."

Tom's physician calculated that his patient was consuming as much as 25 grams of salt a day—an amount that was 10 or 15 times more than Tom needed. He recommended that Tom cut out the excess salt, and not only did Tom's blood pressure fall, it stayed down without the need for drugs of any kind.

Avoiding Something That Can Sneak Up on You

Salt is an essential mineral, and we must have it for normal body function. On the other hand, most Americans eat far too much salt. Studies have shown that the more salt you use on your food, and the saltier the foods that you eat, the greater are your chances of developing high blood pressure. Salt use is a habit, and like most habits it can become such a natural part of your daily life that you don't realize you are in effect poisoning yourself with salt. Excessive use of salt can sneak up on you, and the *high salt intake can contribute to your high blood pressure.*

Blood Pressure Drugs
Work by Eliminating Salt from the Body

Many physicians were skeptical of the value of a low-salt diet in the treatment of high blood pressure. That is, they were skeptical until the introduction of the thiazide diuretics in the early 1960's. So effective are these drugs that most physicians now prescribe them routinely for the treatment of high blood pressure. At first, the blood-pressure-lowering effects of the thiazides weren't understood. Then it became clear that one of the main ways they worked was by causing the patient to lose salt into his urine. In effect, the drug got rid of the excess salt the person had eaten. As the salt left his system, the patient's blood pressure dropped to normal.

Well then, if a pill is available to remove salt from the body, why not take it? For several reasons. The prescriptions are expensive, and so are all those trips to the doctor. One thing eating less salt does is to let you get by on fewer blood pressure pills—or perhaps none at all. Taking fewer pills means running less risk of having a reaction to the drug. The list of ill effects that thiazides can cause is too long to include here, but some of these are stomach and intestinal ulcers, diabetes, gout, kidney damage and a serious form of anemia. Restricting salt is a safer, healthier and less expensive way to lower your blood pressure. Finally, lowering your intake of salt may keep you from getting high blood pressure if you don't already have it.

Putting an Ill-Advised Habit Behind You

Any well-ingrained habit is hard to give up, and you may have convinced yourself that salt is essential to the taste of food. It isn't. Like the appetite for beer or tobacco, the taste for salt is acquired. Children don't want it until the habit is cultivated. Eskimos and another group of people with low salt intake, the Indians of Bolivia, were shown not to like salt when it was first offered, but they very quickly adapted to it. By the same token, persons on a very limited intake of salt do not develop salt craving. And people find that the salt habit is not too hard to give up.

I'm willing to predict that once you stop using salt in excess, you'll never miss it! If anything, you'll enjoy food more, because salt covers up the natural flavor of food. Here are four ways to put this ill advised habit behind you:

(1) Throw away your salt shaker. This is the first step in reducing your salt intake. Stop salting food at the table, and if you have anything to do with preparing meals, do not add salt in cooking—even when the recipe calls for it. Should you worry about not getting enough salt? No! You're going to get more than enough salt from the food that you eat, because all foods contain this mineral. For example, five slices of white bread give you enough salt to supply your body needs for an entire day. Other foods are even saltier, and the saltiest ones should be avoided.

High-Salt Foods*

Vegetables - sauerkraut, pickles and other vegetables prepared in brine

Fruits - olives, maraschino cherries, dried fruit if processed with salt, salted nuts

Breads - bread or rolls with salt topping, potato chips or sticks, corn chips, pretzels, salted popcorn

Cereals - enriched cereals that contain sodium (salt)

Meats - bacon, ham, pork, corned beef, bologna and other luncheon meats, meats made kosher by salting

Beverages - milk, commercial milk products, fountain beverages, sugar-sweetened carbonated beverages, instant cocoa mixes, beer

Spreads - processed cheese, peanut butter, garlic salt, catsup, meat sauces or tenderizers, mustard, onion salt, chili sauce

---

*John G. Deaton, "Stamp Out Salt Pollution," *Life and Health,* October, 1974, p.23. Used by permission of *Life and Health.*

Low-Salt Foods*

Vegetables - fresh cabbage, cucumber, green beans, lettuce, spinach, squash, tomatoes, turnip greens, etc.

Fruits - fresh apples, apricots, bananas, cherries, grapefruit, grapes, oranges, peaches, pineapple, etc.

Breads - bread made without salt, or with sodium-free baking powder

Cereals - unsalted grits, oatmeal, puffed rice, puffed wheat, shredded wheat, etc.

Meats - chicken, beef, lamb, veal, quail, turkey, duck, etc.

Beverages - coffee, fruit juice, tea, alcoholic beverages (except when salt is added), lemonade, etc.

*John G. Deaton, *op. cit.* Used by permission of *Life and Health.*

(2) Do Your Best to Avoid Salty Foods. Take a moment to look at the lists of high-salt foods and low-salt foods. Do your best to cut down on salty foods. For example, pork products such as ham, bacon, sausage and pork chops are just about the saltiest of foods. Cut down on pork products, or eliminate them from your diet entirely. Most seafoods are salty, but you can eat fish if you don't overdo it. Do watch out for salty potatoes and hush puppies. You must also go easy on your intake of high-salt beverages such as beer and milk.

(3) Limit your intake of processed foods. Potato chips, corn chips, salted nuts and snack crackers are loaded with salt. So are such things as TV dinners, pickles and canned items. The salt is a preservative, and the food wouldn't stay fresh without it. In other words, eating processed foods adds to your salt problem.

How Katie W. Learned about Salt Intake the Hard Way

Katie W., a 65-year-old woman, suffered from congestive heart failure. She had recovered from a serious heart attack only to develop heart failure, and her team of physicians was hard put to control the water that collected in her lungs and the swelling that deformed her legs. One way to treat heart failure is to restrict the person's salt intake. This Katie's doctors did, but she continued to have swelling and shortness of breath.

One day I happened by the hospital ward in between rounds and stopped to chat with Katie, who was happily enjoying some saltine crackers. At a pause in the conversation I reminded the patient that she was on a low-salt diet.

"But these are *unsalted* saltines," she protested, pointing to the words on the box. She was right. The crackers were not heavily sprinkled with salt. But they were rich in salt just the same, as it clearly stated on the package label.

Katie gave up her crackers, and her swelling went away.

The lesson? Almost all processed foods contain salt. To take best advantage of a low-salt diet, you have to choose fresh foods over processed foods whenever possible.

(4) Develop a taste for fresh foods. Fresh, natural foods are lowest in salt, and these foods are also the highest in vitamins and other nutrients. When possible, choose them instead of processed foods. Fresh vegetables, fresh fruits and fresh beef can provide a healthy and delicious diet!

The Physician Who Learned of an Active, Drugless Way to Lower Blood Pressure

Physicians are taught to give drugs to treat high blood pressure, but one physician didn't want to take medicine when his own pressure went up. He learned of his high blood pressure at an insurance exam. "I guess you'll have to join the troops taking blood pressure drugs," the examiner said with a chuckle.

"Yes, and it'll probably mean I'll be on them from now on," the physician-patient said. "It's something I don't look forward to."

His wife had an alternate idea. "Why don't you try exercising?" she asked. "I read somewhere that it would lower your blood pressure."

The physician made the excuse that he was too busy to exercise, but later he changed his mind. "You're right," he told his wife. "If I want to avoid taking drugs, I'm going to have to do something else. And it's going to be me that has to do it, not someone doing it for me."

This physician's blood pressure reading had been 160/100 before he started exercising. Six months after he began a program of regular walking and jogging, his blood pressure was down to 138/90. Within a year, his blood pressure was 120/80, and it has not risen far above that level in the five years since then. I'm quite certain of this, because this physician happens to be me! Exercising to lower the blood pressure is a treatment I can vouch for personally.

How Exercise Brings the Blood Pressure Down

The blood pressure reading is a measurement of the amount of force exerted by your heart as it pumps blood into your arteries. As the heart beats, it sends a quantity of blood into the arteries. This blood enters the arteries at a relatively high pressure, known as the "systolic pressure"—the upper reading of the blood pressure. In between each beat of the heart, the pressure drops temporarily, and this lower pressure is the "diastolic pressure"—the lower reading of the blood pressure. Many factors go together to determine what your blood pressure will be.

One of the main things, however, is how easily your blood vessels stretch open to receive the blood pumped into them by your heart. As a rule, the more elastic your vessels, the lower will be your blood pressure. Exercise gives your muscles a workout, but it also helps to keep your vessels young, resilient, and flexible. Another way that exercise lowers your blood pressure is by reminding your body to keep the pressure down. During the actual period of exercise, your blood pressure goes up. Afterward, it goes down by the action of certain reflexes the exercise has brought into play. Exercising regularly keeps these blood-pressure-lowering reflexes working for you.

Deriving Maximum Benefit
from Your Own Activities

The first thing some people want to say when the doctor suggests exercise is, "Oh, I already get enough exercise—just from what I do." Actually, this may not be the case, unless you regularly engage in strenuous activity. By definition, *exercise is that amount of activity you do that is above and beyond the ordinary tasks of the day.* It is an extra dose of walking or running or swimming, and for it to do you the most good you have to exercise every day. Not only that. The activity must be hard enough to make your heart rate go up. You have to work at it, put some effort into it. The nice thing is that the work pays off. Some forms of exercise you can choose are:

- Walking
- Swimming
- Jogging
- Cycling

Any of these exercises, or a combination of them, will help to keep your blood pressure down, provided that you make the exercise a habit and stick with it. Once you have included exercise in your daily activities, you'll find yourself looking forward to this relaxing and pleasant undertaking.

Walking is the exercise most people choose, because it is inexpensive, convenient, readily available—and fun. Some persons will eventually graduate to a mixture of walking and jogging ("jog-walking") or to jogging as the main exercise.

The Thing That Made All the Difference in Reducing Earlene's Blood Pressure

Earlene W., a 49-year-old social worker, had high blood pressure and was overweight. I talked to Earlene about the various ways she could lower her blood pressure, but she requested pills. She left the office with her prescription, only to return two weeks later. "That medicine upsets my stomach." We tried something else, but it gave her diarrhea.

"Earlene," I said, "you're going to have to lose some weight and get started on an exercise program to get your blood pressure down. Not only is that the best way, but in your particular case it may be the only way."

"But I have no time to exercise," she protested. "I work all day and am too tired at night,"

To illustrate how busy she was, Earlene asked me to accompany her to see a client. The client needed a medical examination, and I went along to do it. Riding with Earlene was an experience. We had to stop at three different places before we could locate the client. Parking was a problem, and at each place Earlene would circle the block and continue searching until she had found just the right parking place—one that was very close to the place she was going. When I told her that she sure went to a lot of trouble to avoid walking, Earlene laughed and said, "Yes, people tell me that. I drive my car a block to the store, and one time I took a Gray Lines Tour and wouldn't leave the bus because it was too much trouble to get off and on."

We saw her client, and I performed a medical examination. Then Earlene and I returned to my office. As I was getting out of the car, I said, "Earlene, the best way for you to get your blood pressure down is to sell your car."

Earlene frowned. "I can't do that, but I do see the point you're making. Would it help," she asked, "if I kept my car but tried taking a walk in the mornings, before breakfast?"

"Any walking you do is going to help," I told her. "The more the better." Here is the exercise program she started:

- *A 10-minute walk each morning after breakfast.* Earlene began getting up a little earlier and found that the early morning walk was one of the most peaceful, refreshing times of the day.

- *A 10-minute walk during the lunch hour.* Eating meant a lot to Earlene, but in view of her overweight she began to skimp on her lunch so she would have time to walk at least 10 minutes afterward.

- *A 20-minute walk in the early evening.* Earlene preferred to walk after the evening meal, since the walk served to promote digestion and help her blood pressure at the same time.

As the months passed, Earlene W.'s weight dropped and her blood pressure dropped. When I expressed amazement at how well she had done, she let me in on a little secret. "I'm cheating," she said. "I'm walking more than you prescribed. But the biggest change I've made, the thing that has made the most difference, is in the use of my car. Now I walk to a client's house if the distance is only a mile or so, and I don't spend all that time looking for parking places when I do drive. It occurred to me that I had been acting like a little walking would kill me. From what you said, and from the results I've had from walking, I think the opposite is true. I feel better than I've felt in years, and I think walking is responsible."

Five Steps to Your Own Blood-Pressure-Lowering Activity

If you have high blood pressure and perhaps are overweight, a regular walking program can mean as much to you as it did to Earlene. Here are the five steps you can use to set up your own blood-pressure-lowering activity:

STEP ONE: BEGIN WITH A CHECK-UP

The first step for anyone just starting an exercise program is a medical check-up. Discuss with your doctor what you plan to do, and get the physician's opinion. Unless you have heart disease or some other limitation—and even heart disease need not be a limitation in all cases—your doctor will no doubt roundly endorse your exercise program. And the physician will continue to follow you to evaluate the blood-pressure-lowering effects of exercise.

STEP TWO: MAKE IT YOUR PERSONAL PROGRAM

Your exercise program is for YOU! If you wish to do calisthenics with a group, do so. But don't fall into the trap of thinking that you have to have a group to exercise. The very best exercise program is one that you develop and do by yourself.

How Mrs. B. Learned That Personal Exercise Is Easy Exercise

Mrs. B., a 56-year-old patient of mine, began exercising regularly at the Y. Her blood pressure began to fall and things were looking good, but then she stopped going to the sessions. I asked her what had happened.

"I was doing fine, but then my exercise group at the Y lost its instructor. They disbanded the group until they could locate another instructor. It's been two months, and I haven't done any exercise since then."

This patient would not have had this problem if she had taken up her own, personal exercise program right from the start. At my urging, she began to walk for fifteen minutes three times a day, and she found that she liked that much better than fighting the traffic to go to the Y. "Now," she told me a few months later when her blood pressure had started down again, "I can exercise during the time I used to spend driving to the Y. It's so much easier, so much better. I can exercise when I want to and where I want to."

STEP THREE: START SLOWLY AND WORK YOUR WAY UP

Many people learn the hard way that any exercise program must be one of starting slowly and building up gradually. Starting too quickly can cause you to have soreness and stiffness in your muscles the following day. You may want to try walking for five minutes at a time the first week and then gradually work up to walking 15 minutes at a time, three times a day. Do these muscle-stretching exercises before you begin walking:

• *Hamstring stretchers.* The hamstrings are a group of muscles at the back of each thigh. Stretch them by sitting with one leg or the other straight out in front of you. Reach toward the toes of this leg, and you will feel a tightening in the back of your thigh. Do the exercise about five times and perform hamstring stretching on the opposite leg, after first repositioning yourself. Don't worry if you can't touch your toes to begin with. Just reaching toward them will stretch the hamstrings.

• *Calf stretchers.* Stand about two or three feet from a wall; you may need to stand four feet away if you are above average height. Fall toward the wall and catch yourself with your hands. Your heels will lift as you do this. Now, return your heels to the floor and hold them down for a count of five or ten. Then raise your heels and lower them again for a count of five. Repeat the exercise several times. As your muscles get unlimbered you'll find that you have to stand a little farther away from the wall to stretch the calf muscles. This is natural and simply means that your legs are in much better shape than when you started.

• *Abdominal strengtheners.* Lie flat on your back with your hands beneath your buttocks. Take in a breath, hold it, and lift your feet into the air. If your tummy is large and you are out of shape, you may not be able to get your feet more than a few inches off the ground. Nevertheless, attempt to do so: Lift your feet as far as you can without undue exertion, let them down, and repeat the exercise five times. Another way to srengthen the abdominals is to do sit-ups. However, sit-ups are not as safe as the exercise just described, and you probably shouldn't do them unless you're used to them and know they won't hurt your back. The important thing is to tighten those tummy muscles by getting your feet into the air. An added benefit of abdominal strengtheners is that they will cause your waistline to shrink.

STEP FOUR: WEAR WHAT IS COMFORTABLE

The beauty of walking is that it requires no special uniform! Wear comfortable, loose-fitting clothing. Obviously, you are going to need to wrap up when the weather is cold, and in the heat of the summer you may find it enjoyable to wear shorts and a pullover of cotton or jersey.

Shoes? The ones that feel good on your feet. Any low-quarter, comfortable shoe will do to walk in, but purchase tennis or jogging shoes if you wish.

If you are subject to blisters on your feet when you walk, here's a way to avoid them. *Wear two pairs of socks.* Put on a regular pair of close-fitting nylon socks and then over them wear thick wool or cotton socks. This way, motion can occur between the two socks rather than between the sock and your skin. Fewer blisters.

STEP FIVE: TURN YOUR WALKING INTO FUN!

Integrate your exercise program with your other activities. Never ride when you can walk! Move around on foot and discover what you've been missing when you drove past in your car. Hoof it, and an entire new world will open to you!

Remember, for example, how falling leaves rustle in an autumn wind? In the autumn it is a lovely thing to glide beneath tall trees and feel the leaves crunch beneath your feet. Ever notice how grease spots on a road turn into individual rainbows when the sun first peeks out after a shower? You can see this when you begin walking. How long has it been since you pulled off your shoes and felt moist earth beneath your toes? On a warm spring walk there is nothing more delightful! You'll meet others who themselves are out walking, you'll feel better and you'll lower your blood pressure at the same time.

We'll take up some additional details of your walking program in the next chapter, *Boosting Your Vitality by Keeping Your Heart and Vessels Young.*

How George Learned an Important Blood-Pressure-Lowering Secret

George was a driving, energetic man of 50. He owned a business, and he was not going to let high blood pressure slow him down. He took his blood pressure pills on the run, and he was disappointed that the medicine didn't work the way it was supposed to. George saw several physicians because of his elevated blood pressure, and by the time he got to me he was discouraged. "I just don't think anything will work for me," he said.

"There may be one thing," I told him. "You may be able to work for yourself."

"How?"

"Well, to start with you're going to have to reduce the amount of stress that you are under. You're driving yourself too hard, and that's probably helping to cause your blood pressure to go up. You're going to have to take it easier."

"Impossible!" was his brisk reply. "I've built my business with my own two hands. No way I'm going to let go of it." He explained that his firm was in a head-to-head struggle with another firm to land a huge government contract. "There's more than just the money involved," George confided. "That other company is owned by a boy I went to high school with. We used to date the same girl, played on the same team. We've been after each other all our lives, and most of the time he's got the best of me. No, doctor, I can't slow down now. Just give me some pills and I'll see you in a month. Right now I'm going out and getting that contract. It means too much to me to lose."

"George," I cautioned, "you don't have a choice in this. You're headed for a stroke or a heart attack unless you slow down."

He left in a huff. Two days later he phoned me from his office. He sounded like a changed man. "Doctor, you were right, " he said. "Things were going to heck down here, and me right in the thick of it. Then I got a telephone call that really shook me up. Now I'm ready to come back and see if you can help me slow down. I promise to follow your advice to the letter."

"What was the call about?"

"You remember me telling you about the guy I went to high school with, who owns the company I'm competing with? His wife said he just dropped dead of a stroke. He was going at the same pace as me, but it may not be too late if I do something beginning right now."

George did ease up, and it did him a world of good. He hired some assistants to do things he used to do, and he found that relaxing for easy power did more than just lower his blood pressure. It made him a better businessman. His firm also managed to get that government contract.

Taking the Time
to Handle Stress in a Healthy Manner

Stress, worry, tension—these are three things that we almost seem to accept as a part of modern living. But they needn't be. Merely taking the time to cope with stress in a healthy manner can mean the difference between having a normal blood pressure and having an elevated one.

When you let tension get the best of you, it acts on your nervous system to cause your blood pressure to go up. One medicine that is commonly used to lower the blood pressure is phenobarbital—a tranquilizer. But you can be your own tranquilizer by reacting to problems in a tension-free way. Here are some tips on how to do this:

• *Make relaxing a habit.* Find a quiet place at least three times a day. Sit back in a comfortable chair and let your body go limp. Allow your mind to be at ease. Think pleasant thoughts, perhaps of something that you are looking forward to doing. Spend five minutes in complete relaxation, and you'll be able to feel the tension easing out of your shoulders and back and arms and legs. As relaxing becomes a habit, you'll find that your feeling of calm and confidence carries into the other parts of the day.

• *Take a load off your mind.* If you are in a position to do so, delegate authority to subordinates. The person who benefits most from the relief of stress is the driving, energetic person who believes that nothing will get done unless he himself does it. Don't carry the world on your shoulders, because it's far too heavy! Let your associates share some of the load. Doing so will make you feel better, and it will make them feel better, too. Difficult problems should be discussed openly with someone. Just the simple act of unloading your problems to an intimate—and hearing that person out—will go a long way toward the relief of tension.

• *Use the secrets of the calm people.* A lovely white-haired lady, a nurse, once told me that she did not let herself get too upset with things, because she knew the effect it could have. "I try to be tactful with other people and show them that I care. Whatever I do, I try to remain relaxed. I've made it a habit not to say things in anger and to be courteous even when others are discourteous. And you know, it works. But the best way I've found to head off tension is to have a good time. As long as I am enjoying myself, I'm relaxed. I try to fill each day with many pleasant things, and I look forward to them one at a time. A happy life is a relaxed life."

Relax, and you'll learn to benefit from happiness and contentment.

How Eldon Gave Up One Thing and Got Two Things in Return

Eldon, a 62-year-old farmer, developed coldness and tingling in his feet. His feet felt numb after he had been walking for several minutes, and he complained of pain in his calves when he walked. Physicians diagnosed the problem as a disease of the blood vessels to Eldon's legs. They were alarmed about two things: Eldon had high blood pressure, and he smoked two packs of cigarettes a day.

"We may have to operate on your leg arteries," the surgeon said, "but it would be a lot better if you gave up smoking first. Cigarettes contain a drug that cuts down on your circulation. Stop smoking, and your legs'll do a lot better."

Eldon went home to consider the doctors' advice. His wife had been after him to stop smoking, but he hadn't listened. For him, smoking was just a habit, a 40-year habit, nothing he considered was actually hurting him. He lit a cigarette and ambled down to the barn behind the house. He had to stop and rest about every ten yards. Suddenly he grew angry with himself. He threw the cigarette down and ground it out with his heel. He clenched his fists and vowed to never smoke another.

His improvement was gradual. His doctors put him on a program of exercise, and the surgeon was hopeful that the operation could be delayed. His giving up smoking helped Eldon in another way. His blood pressure dropped so that he didn't have to take as many pills as previously.

"If I'd known it would do this much for me," the farmer told me, "I'd have quit smoking long ago."

The Single Act That Can Mean So Much

Quitting smoking can improve your health in so many ways! We'll be discussing some of these in other parts of this book. But if you smoke and have high blood pressure, you can definitely expect your pressure to go down when you stop smoking. Give up this habit, and you'll need less blood pressure medicine.

Probably the Most Important Thing You Can Do

Probably the most important thing you can do for high blood pressure, provided you are overweight, is to lose weight! Losing weight is the subject of a separate chapter, *Staying Young by Losing Pounds the Natural Way*. Reduce to your ideal weight, and your blood pressure may return to normal without the need for drugs. And that's only one of the things losing weight will do for you! (See Chapter 6.)

How All These Things Work Together to Help You

As we will discuss in the chapter on weight loss, exercise is an excellent way to burn calories and thus shed pounds. Losing weight helps to lower your blood pressure. So does the exercise itself. And exercise, especially when the weather is hot, makes you perspire. Perspiration removes salt from your body. As salt leaves your system, your blood pressure goes down. Finally, people who care enough about their good health to exercise and eat a low-salt diet and lose weight are not going to lose all these good benefits by continuing to smoke. In other words, once you begin lowering your blood pressure the drugless way, you'll find that all things discussed in this chapter work together to help your blood pressure go down more quickly.

Knowing When Your Pressure Is Normal and When It Isn't

The so-called "normal" blood pressure usually listed in health books is *120/80*. The systolic reading is 120, and the diastolic reading is 80. Yes, 120/80 is a normal blood pressure, but it is only an *average* reading. Your blood pressure could be 135/70, or 128/85, or 140/90, and it would still be normal. Almost any blood pressure below 140/90 is normal. Pressures between 140/90 and 150/100 are borderline, and pressures above 150/100 are definitely high.

Some people get the notion that the blood pressure is only one number. Patients tell me, "My pressure was one-sixty," or, "The doctor said my pressure was a hundred and fifty." A person who says this is referring to his *systolic blood pressure*—the upper reading that corresponds to the beat of the heart. The lower reading, the *diastolic blood pressure*, occurs in between heartbeats; it is actually the more important of the two readings.

The drugless ways of lowering the blood pressure discussed in this chapter will lower both the systolic and the diastolic readings.

How to Take Your Own Blood Pressure

Many a person finds it convenient and desirable to take his own blood pressure at home, or to have his spouse take it. Learning to take your blood pressure is not difficult. Here's what you do:

• *Obtain the equipment.* You need two things: an ordinary stethoscope and the pressure-recording apparatus, known by the tongue-twisting name of sphygmomanometer, or *sphygmo* for short. You can purchase a stethoscope and a sphygmo at a medical supply store, in surplus stores, or even in department stores.

• *Prepare for the exam.* Have the "patient" sit comfortably or lie down. Wrap the cuff of the sphygmo around the person's upper arm and secure it snugly. (It makes no difference which arm you choose.) Fit the stethoscope into your ears, taking care that the angulated earpieces point forward, toward your eyes. Place the listening end of the stethoscope at the crook of the person's arm, just below the lower edge of the sphygmo cuff.

• *Inflate the cuff.* Inflate the sphygmo cuff until the attached pressure gage records a reading of about 200. Then, while listening with the stethoscope, slowly let the air out of the cuff. By raising the pressure in the cuff to 200, you shut off the flow of blood through the main artery in the person's arm. Now that you are letting the air out of the cuff, the blood will begin to flow into the arm once again. You will be able to hear it start to do so as you listen through the stethoscope. A caution: Let the air out of the cuff fairly slowly. A rate of about 2 mm. a second is just right.

• *Record the systolic pressure.* The systolic, or upper, pressure reading will be announced by a sharp click or bump. You'll hear this sound and a series of continuing bump-bump-bumps. The first "bump" is the important one. Note the pressure in the gage when you hear it. Remember this reading, because it is the systolic blood pressure.

• *Record the diastolic pressure.* The clicking or bumping sounds will get softer and softer and will finally disappear. Continue to look at the pressure gage and note the pressure when you can no longer hear any clicking sounds through the stethoscope. The reading on the gage when the clicking sounds disappear represents the diastolic pressure.

• *Write the pressure down.* Always keep a record of your blood pressure readings. They are valuable for your own records and for use by your doctor, who will want to know what the readings have been at home. (Most physicians do not object to a patient taking his own blood pressure. In fact, many physicians request their patients to do this.) The standard way to write the blood pressure is with the systolic reading as the numerator and the diastolic reading as the denominator. Commonly, the two numbers are separated by a slash: 120/80.

You don't need to take your pressure more often than about once a week, and you should take it at a time when you have been relaxing for an hour or so. Following your own pressure can be fun, especially when you are able to see the benefits of your blood-pressure-lowering efforts.

5

Boosting Your Vitality by Keeping Your Heart and Vessels Young

You've seen people who go through life bubbling with energy. They greet each day with the freshness and excitement of a ten-year-old. They are happy, active people, because they have learned that the secret of keeping young is to keep your heart and vessels that way. By making the conscious effort to have a healthy heart and healthy vessels, you can share this secret and boost your own vitality! The blood vessels are the highways of the body, and the heart sends health-giving nutrients down these highways to every part of you. The better your circulation works, the more vitality you'll have. And the greater your vitality, the better you'll feel. In fact, you're as young as your heart and vessels! The five ways to keep your heart and vessels young are:

1. *Begin to do something now, not later!*
2. *Eat sensibly by avoiding high-fat foods.*
3. *Make exercise a part of your life.*
4. *Stop smoking (or don't start).*
5. *Lose weight if you are overweight.*

The Day Jack C. Learned the Truth about Heart Disease

I dreaded Jack's visits! He would drop into the examining room looking much older than his 48 years, and he was never able to smile or exchange pleasantries. The day I am remembering started no differently from usual. Jack took a seat next to the desk, hauled out his medicines from a paper sack, and looked at me. He tried to hold eye contact for as long as possible, and written all over his face was a plea for help. He seemed to be saying "Help me, doctor. Please help me. Unless you do something for me, I am going to die."

Only a few months earlier, Jack had been sailing along in apparent good health. He operated a dry-cleaning business, worked long hours and enjoyed life. I was on duty at the hospital when an ambulance brought him in one night about ten o'clock. He had eaten dinner at the usual hour, sat down in front of the television to relax with the paper, and begun to have indigestion. Over the next few hours the "indigestion" became a steady ache, like "somebody was pushing his fist against my breastbone." Then the pain began to move down Jack's left shoulder to his elbow. He broke out in a sweat. My examination and the electrocardiogram confirmed that Jack C. had suffered a heart attack, a bad one. His hospital stay was stormy. Twice he nearly died when his heart stopped beating, and he had to fight his way through the frightening experience of water-logged lungs—a complication of his weak heart. Jack had been out of the hospital for three months, but hadn't returned to work. He hadn't done much of anything, in fact, because he still thought that he was going to die.

"Your medical progress has been very good, Jack," I told him on this particular day. "The electrocardiogram still shows a scar, but there are no signs of new activity, and your pain hasn't returned."

The patient just stared at me.

"Jack," I said, feeling the blood rush to my face because I was saying something that perhaps I shouldn't say, "you're not going to die! You're going to get well."

He began crying. As he cried he told me the things I already knew. That he had always been in good health. That he hadn't had to watch what he ate. That he had let himself get overweight, but what was wrong with that?

Quietly and with what I hoped was compassion, I explained to Jack that his heart disease had not suddenly developed the night of his heart attack. By what he ate, by his lack of exercise, by the way he lived, Jack had been setting himself up for a heart attack for at least 30 years.

The Most Important Lesson Is the Easiest One to Forget

Jack had made the mistake so many people make. He had presumed because he'd never had a heart attack that his heart and blood vessels were normal. It just doesn't work that way! Heart disease develops slowly, and its rate of progress is influenced by almost everything you do. By "heart disease" I mean blockage of the coronary arteries, the pencil-sized vessels that carry blood to the heart muscle itself. Heart disease and blood vessel disease cause over one-half of the deaths in the United States each year, and chemical analysis of the sludge that causes coronary blockage has shown that it consists of saturated fats and cholesterol.

The important lesson here is that the time to start doing something about the build-up of sludge in the coronary arteries is NOW! Autopsies of American soldiers killed in combat during the Korean War showed that three-fourths of young men in their late teens and early twenties already had significant coronary atherosclerosis. Over the years the disease progresses until it becomes severe enough to cause a heart attack.

Prevention is the best treatment for heart disease, but if you are like Jack and already have heart trouble, the same methods that work to keep the heart and vessels in peak condition can also work to return your heart to its best possible efficiency. In fact, once Jack C. understood that healthy living was as important to him as the heart pills, his entire outlook changed. By beginning to do things for himself in a positive way, he overcame his fear of death and took the major role in his own treatment. One day as he was leaving the office he said, "Doc, I appreciate so much what you've told me. I know I'm on top of this heart disease now. But I'd give just about anything if I'd had the sense to start this program *before* I had a heart attack."

How the Healthy Way to a Man's Heart Can Be through His Stomach

What you eat does matter! It matters to men and women both, though men are more likely to get heart disease and vascular disease than women. Doctors aren't sure why. Apparently, a woman's natural blood chemicals protect her heart. However, this effect lasts only so long as she continues to have menstrual cycles. After the age of 50 or 60, a woman's risk of developing heart disease becomes as great as the risk of a man her age.

The circumstantial evidence linking a fatty diet to heart disease is overwhelming, though scientists haven't yet worked out all the details on how the fat gets from your stomach into your heart. To use a comparison, let's speak of snakebite. We knew that the bite of a king cobra was fatal long before we could say that the victim's quick death was due to a poisonous neurotoxin contained in the venom injected by the snake. We don't have to know *how* a high-fat diet kills somebody before taking steps to avoid fatty poisons!

Sensible eating means avoiding foods that are high in saturated fats. You can do this by following these rules:

> *Rule 1. Switch to low-fat milk.*
>
> *Rule 2. Use margarine instead of butter.*
>
> *Rule 3. Select your breakfast foods carefully.*
>
> *Rule 4. Avoid fatty traps.*
>
> *Rule 5. Cook sensibly.*

RULE 1. SWITCH TO LOW-FAT MILK

Milk is proclaimed by its advertisers to be "nature's most nearly perfect food." No doubt milk is nutritious. However, just because something is nutritious doesn't mean that large quantities of it are necessarily good for you. Even relatively small amounts of whole milk, consumed every day for a lifetime, can be damaging to your heart and vessels. And certain milk products, such as butter, buttermilk, cream and cheese, are loaded with saturated fats.

What is a *saturated* fat? The word "saturated" describes a particular chemical pattern in the fat molecule. Saturated fats come from an animal source, such as the cow, the hog or the chicken. Fats derived from vegetables have a particular chemical pattern that is called *unsaturated*. Studies have shown that saturated fats, including cholesterol, are what pile up in your arteries to cause heart disease and other circulatory conditions. Unsaturated fats, however, have the opposite effect. They may actually protect against the deposition of saturated fats in the arteries. The point to remember is that *sensible eating means taking in as few saturated fats as possible.* Switching from whole milk to low-fat milk is one way of doing this.

Here are the advantages of drinking low-fat milk:

- *It is less expensive than whole milk.*
- *It contains up to 99% fewer saturated fats than whole milk.*
- *It contains far fewer calories than whole milk.*
- *In spite of its low fat content, it still is fortified with vitamins D and E.*
- *It tastes great!* In fact, once you've gotten used to the taste of low-fat milk, regular milk by comparison will taste fatty and unpleasant.

To enjoy good health, children need a glass of milk a day, but they can get all the nutrients they need from low-fat milk. Be sure to use low-fat milk instead of cream in cereal, coffee or tea, and give up buttermilk completely. It's also a good idea to choose low-fat cheese and low-fat ice cream (ice milk), though you can be reasonable about this. Several helpings a week of regular cheese or ice cream won't hurt you. Fatty foods eaten day after day at every meal will.

RULE 2. USE MARGARINE INSTEAD OF BUTTER

Not long ago my wife and I were dining out, and the waiter brought us some little packets of yellow to use on our rolls. "Is this margarine or butter?" I asked. The waiter looked offended. "It's *butter*, sir," he said, as if to serve anything else would have been cheap and contemptible. He was shocked when I asked him to return his butter to the kitchen and bring me some margarine.

Certain food practices have gotten ingrained into our thinking, and changing them takes a lot of effort. Why margarine? Because most margarines are made of vegetable oils and thus contain unsaturated fats. Butter, by contrast, is 100% saturated fat. Bad for the heart and vessels.

Incidentally, margarine made from unsaturated vegetable oils such as corn oil works just as well as butter in recipes, and you can find other uses for it as well. My wife taught me how to cook pinto beans, and one of the steps was to add a piece of fatty ham to give flavor to the slowly simmering pot of beans. Once when I had no ham I decided to put margarine into the pot instead. It worked perfectly! The beans tasted great, and we had exchanged the unsaturated fat of margarine for the saturated fat of ham.

RULE 3. SELECT YOUR BREAKFAST FOODS CAREFULLY.

The usual breakfast foods—eggs, ham, bacon and sausage—are high in saturated fats. Far from being "health-giving" or "energy-providing," these breakfast foods can load your system with fats and speed you on your way to heart disease. You may know of someone who ate these foods every morning and lived to be a hundred. Fine. But that might be a quirk. Heart disease is caused by the interaction of many different factors: your diet, your activity, your blood pressure and your inherited tendency to develop fatty plaques in your vessels. Unless you know for sure that you are immune from heart disease, you should select your breakfast foods carefully.

How Lonnie Learned to Start the Day the Right Way

His name was Lonnie, and he was only 26 years old. He was a sergeant in the Army, he was overweight, and he had one of the worst heart attacks I had ever seen. The attack injured every part of Lonnie's heart, and I feared for his life. Lonnie survived, probably because of his youth, and during his weeks of recuperation I had the chance to take a detailed dietary history.

My patient had grown up on a farm in Wisconsin, and he started each day with a huge breakfast. He drank two glasses of whole milk or buttermilk, he spread a thick helping of butter or cheese on his bread, and he downed generous portions of eggs and ham and sausage. "Breakfast is the most important meal of the day," Lonnie told me, but I had something to tell him.

"Your problem is that you've been eating the wrong breakfast. You've been loading yourself up with that high-fat stuff, and I'm convinced it's what's built up in your coronary vessels and caused your heart attack. First thing you're going to need to do is switch to low-fat milk and get off of butter. And then you're going to have to start eating a sensible breakfast."

The things I told Lonnie to avoid, and which I would recommend that everyone stay away from, are:

Breakfast Foods to Avoid:
- Eggs
- Sausage
- Ham
- Bacon
- Butter, whole milk, buttermilk, and cream

What You Hear May Not Necessarily Be True

In the Southwest as well as in other parts of the country, a popular country singer advertises his own brand of sausage. He talks about how important it is to eat a "good old country breakfast" and even goes so far as to imply that sausage is good for you. This is absurd!

Sausage, like bacon and eggs, is loaded with saturated fats. These fats may taste good, and they may stick to your ribs so that you don't get hungry until lunch, but they are anything but good for you. Their high content of saturated fats means that they are BAD FOR YOUR HEART AND VESSELS. The best policy is to stay away from sausage, ham and bacon. Eggs? The white of an egg is protein, and won't hurt your heart at all. But the yellow of an egg ranks number one as the most highly concentrated food source of cholesterol! For the sake of your heart, limit yourself to no more than one or two eggs a week. And remember, you're probably getting eggs in some of the lunch and supper dishes you eat.

Breakfast Foods That Are Okay:
- Cold cereals
- Oatmeal
- Cream of wheat
- Hominy grits
- Cream of rice
- Toast

- Biscuits made from low-fat ingredients
- Juice, coffee, tea
- Sausage and egg substitutes (These contain no saturated fats and can be purchased at the frozen foods counter.)

How Sherry Learned the Benefits of a Cereal Breakfast

Sherry, a 34-year-old housewife, enjoyed good health. She never drank milk or ate sausage or eggs, but this was simply because she didn't like these things. She did fix a piping hot breakfast for her husband and children. Her husband Jim, a 44-year-old college professor, was overweight. He preferred reading to exercising, and he ate whatever happened to be on the table. Jim began to have chest pains when he strode from his office to the lecture room, and a medical evaluation revealed that his cholesterol count was about twice as high as it should have been.

As part of Jim's treatment, his doctor put him on a low-cholesterol diet. Eggs were out. Sausage was out. Butter was out. Whole milk was out. Sherry began to fix cereal for breakfast, to the discontent of her husband and two children. The eaters didn't like going without foods they had grown used to, but they stuck with the new diet.

Three months later, Jim was surprised and pleased to hear that his cholesterol level had fallen to a normal range. His chest pain had also lessened. He told his wife the good news, and she suggested a big hot breakfast as a celebration. Jim shook his head. "Nope! To tell the truth I do feel better not eating that heavy stuff, and I'm staying away from it. Besides, I've gotten to like cereal." The interesting thing was that the children had come to feel the same way. Sherry had developed her own eating habits as a matter of preference, but it wasn't until her husband had his problem with high cholesterol that she understood the true goodness of a cereal breakfast.

RULE 4: AVOID FATTY TRAPS.

It's impossible to totally exclude fat from your diet, and it isn't necessary. Most foods contain a mixture of carbohydrates, proteins and fats. But some foods are much higher in fat than others, and you should take pains to avoid these fatty traps. Some tips:

1. *Choose beef or poultry rather than pork.* Ham, pork chops and sausage are higher in fat content than lean beef, chicken or turkey. Plan your menus around low-fat items, and remember that fish is both delicious and low in fat content.

2. *Select **high-quality ground beef.*** Surveys indicate that ground beef is the most commonly used meat in America. This is fine, because hamburger meat is delicious. By paying a little more, however, you can purchase ground meat that is very low in fat content. Lean ground beef is sometimes labeled "ground round" or "ground chuck." If in doubt, ask the butcher. If you are fortunate to have your own stock (or side of beef), ask the butcher to grind up some of the leanest cuts, first trimming them of all visible fat, and use this lean beef for your hamburger meat. On a volume basis, less of the low-fat ground beef melts away during cooking. And the meat that gets into your mouth contains less fat and cholesterol to reach your vessels and cause fatty plaques.

3. *Choose pressed beef or pressed chicken instead of cold cuts.* Thinly cut slices of chicken or beef are much lower in fat content than widely used cold cuts such as bologna, liverwurst or pastrami. Frankfurters, often advertised as "high in beef," are anything but. Most of any wiener is saturated fat, and you and your family would be better off eating peanut butter. Peanut butter is just as high in calories, but much lower in saturated fats.

4. *Eat fruits for dessert when possible.* Pies, cakes and doughnuts are delectable, right? They're also high in fats and usually contain eggs and butter. Pastries you buy in a store or at a restaurant are especially bad. Why? Because most bakeries cook with shortening made from animal fats. This shortening is cheaper than unsaturated cooking oil—and far more dangerous to your heart. Make your dessert an apple, banana, orange, peach or pear. Try adding fruit cocktail to fresh fruits and top with diced coconut, strawberries, or non-diary whipped topping, which contains no saturated fats.

RULE 5: COOK SENSIBLY.

How you cook food is as important as what you eat. The best way to prepare meat is in a way that will remove most of its fat before it reaches the table. Here are the tips:

1. *Trim the meat before you cook it.* Gourmets beware! The more expensive the cut of meat, the more fat it contains. Those white streaks in raw steak, the marbling, represent fat deposits. You're better off to select meat with the least marbling! And you should trim away all visible fat from the edges and other parts of the meat that is served you at the table. Cutting visible fat off of meat is one of the easiest ways to protect yourself from heart disease.

The Man Who Turned Sensible Eating to His Advantage in His Fight against Heart Disease

Dick was a laboratory technologist, and he met me for lunch one day in the hospital cafeteria. The meat served in the cafeteria that day was a fatty, greasy kind of roast beef (yes, I said it was a *hospital* cafeteria). Dick and I were discussing an article, and my mind was on writing rather than eating. But I couldn't help noticing that my companion not only dug into his food with relish, he ate the fatty part of the roast beef as well as the lean. We had lunch again a few weeks later, and the same thing happened, only this time the fare was pork chops. Dick cleaned the bones. Toward the end of the meal I saw him reach for some small white tablets and put one under his tongue.

I asked him if he had chest pain.

"Nothing, just some angina pectoris."

Angina pectoris is not the same as a heart attack, but it is definitely a sign of heart disease. It had been present for almost a year, Dick said, and the nitroglycerin tablets had been prescribed by a heart specialist. The thing that alarmed me was that Dick was still eating wrong.

"Those nitro tablets may relieve your pain," I told him, "but they do nothing for the fat deposits that are already in your arteries. And believe me, eating fat the way you do is only making the situation worse."

Next time I saw Dick, he rushed over to shake my hand. "Say, I told my doctor what you said, and he agreed completely. He said the reason he doesn't emphasize the dietary treatment of heart disease is that most people don't want to go to the trouble to stick to a diet. But he put me on one and I'm darned if I don't think I'm having less pain than I used to have. And doctor, if what I eat can help my heart, I'm all for it."

2. *Bake or broil instead of frying.* Figure that frying a food will increase its caloric content by at least a third. One way to get around frying potatoes or seafood is to buy these items precooked in the frozen foods counter. They have been fried before you buy them, but are usually not too greasy after you warm them in the oven. Better yet, buy your own potatoes and bake them! Just don't load the baked potato up with cream cheese or sour cream or butter. A little margarine will do nicely. When it becomes necessary to fry something, use corn oil or soybean oil instead of cooking grease.

3. *Discard the drippings from meat.* Make sure that your broiler or baking pan is positioned so that the run-offs from sizzling meat can flow away. Do not collect the fatty drippings to make gravy! Do not collect the fatty drippings to make anything! Throw the fat out!

Eating and cooking sensibly mean, simply, that you take your heart into consideration when you eat. It's not too hard. In the first place, you don't have to give up everything you like and carry on about how bad eating it could be for your heart. But do remember to eat and cook sensibly. What matters most is the track record that you build up over the years.

Taking Advantage of the Two Body Parts
Brenda Used in Her Winning
Fight against Heart Failure

Brenda W., a 60-year-old retired vocational nurse, got sick while on vacation. She and her husband made their home in Chicago and were on their way to Estes Park in Colorado when Brenda developed fever, chest pain and shortness of breath. They stopped in a small town where a physician diagnosed the flu and said that it shouldn't interfere with the vacation. However, Brenda's husband wasn't so sure. After watching his wife in a motel for a day, he put her in the car and drove back to Illinois.

It was a good thing he did. Tests showed that Brenda had myocarditis, a rare but serious infection of the heart muscle; a physician put her in the hospital. Her difficulty in breathing was due to heart failure, and she was bothered by painful swelling of her feet and ankles.

Treatment included digitalis, diuretics, low-salt diet and bed rest. Brenda responded and was able to go home after four weeks. By then she could breathe much better, but the swelling in her legs persisted. Her natural inclination was to take it easy, to move around as little as possible.

Her physician had other ideas. He told her that her heart muscle had been damaged by the viral infection, but that the infection was over. Chances were good that she could recover her health more quickly if she were a little more active. Jogging or cycling wasn't indicated, but walking wouldn't hurt her if she did it in small quantities. "You're a nurse, Brenda, and you know the value of rehabilitation. Rest is excellent treatment so far as it goes, but now it's time to use two of your body parts to get to feeling better. The two body parts are your right leg and your left."

The doctor wrote Brenda an exercise prescription, which she faithfully followed. The swelling in her legs was slow to leave, but because she took her medicine and faithfully followed the exercise program, she and her husband were able to take their vacation to Colorado the following summer.

How You Benefit from Keeping the World's Most Fantastic Pump in Tip-Top Shape

The heart is a muscle, and it pumps blood. It has no other function, and yet it is just as essential to thinking as is the brain, to digestion as are the intestines, and to walking as are the legs. Your heart beats one hundred thousand times a day and forty million times a year! Each day it pumps six tons of blood through more than sixty thousand miles of the circulatory system! The work it does is equal to lifting a ten-pound weight three feet off the ground twice a minute for every hour of your life!

The heart is the world's most fantastic pump, and the way you can keep it in tip-top shape is by exercising it. Again, exercise is the amount of activity you do that is over and above your ordinary routine. The heart needs this extra work to stay strong or to help it recover its strength after a heart attack or other ailment. Of course, if you have ever had heart disease, do not begin an exercise program without first checking with your physician. Follow an exercise program only under a physician's guidance. The benefits you can expect from regular exercise include:

- *Better circulation.* Exercise stimulates the body to grow bigger and better blood vessels.

- *A stronger heart.* Exercise invigorates the heart and sends more blood pumping to the heart muscle.

- *Improved lung function.* The heavy breathing you do during exercise helps your lungs to work better, and the good effects of this stay with you during the rest of the day.

- *A higher blood count.* Exercise infuses new cells into your bloodstream and sets the body to making more red blood cells.

- *Weight reduction.* Exercise not only causes you to lose weight, it can help to lower the fat levels in your blood. On the other hand, if you do not need to lose weight, exercise will tone up your heart and muscles and allow you to eat more without gaining weight.

How Bob Discovered the Right Way
and the Wrong Way to Exercise

Bob was not one of my patients, but I used to see him from time to time on the golf course. As was true for many men, Bob's only "exercise" was golf. However, he didn't walk from green to green; he rode. "Heck," he told me with a chuckle, "worst thing about playing golf was the walking. Now I got this cart I don't have to."

Bob had a heart attack, and while he was recovering his doctor gave him some advice. "Bob," the physician said, "you're soft. You've fallen victim to the American way. You don't walk, you ride. You don't mow your yard, you sit down and ride over it. You use power lawn trimmers, power hedge clippers. You use an electric knife, an electric can opener, an electric toothbrush and electric scissors. You consider automatic clotheswashers and clothesdryers and dishwashers a necessity, and you told me you couldn't get around a golf course without your golf cart. What you and all of us are doing is depriving the heart of the thing it needs most: exercise."

Bob began to think about this, and he saw that the physician was right. Best of all, he made up his mind to do something about his lack of exercise. I don't play golf anymore, and neither does Bob. But I still see him from time to time. I pass him on the hike-and-bike hill country trails nearby. He has become an avid walker. He's lost weight, his heart seems to be in good shape, and he feels better than he has in years. The program that Bob developed is one I would recommend to everyone. Here are the simple steps:

- *Walk every day.*
- *Try to walk an hour, either all at once or in two or three walking sessions during the day.*
- *Set a walking pace of about one mile in 15 minutes, or four miles an hour.*

Making Best Use of Your Own Program

We began the discussion of your personal exercise program in the previous chapter. Once you've learned the unlimbering exercises and begun to walk slowly for short distances, you're ready to advance to the next gradation of exercise. Use your car's speedometer (or odometer) to lay out a one-mile course near your home or some place where you can exercise. Time yourself to see how long it takes to walk this mile. If it takes about 15 minutes, you're right on the mark. If it takes you 20 minutes to go a mile, don't fret. Just let doing a 15-minute mile be your goal. Beyond that, your eventual goal is to walk two, three or four miles each day and to walk them at the speed of four miles an hour. Of course, after you've learned the pace of a 15-minute mile, you don't need to restrict yourself to the one-mile course. You'll know the right speed, and you can concentrate on enjoying the walk, whether it's through a park, a neighborhood, along a river bank or down a country road.

Some people like to go further than four miles, while others prefer to go half this distance. The amount of exercise you do depends on you, and on your doctor's advice. One thing is certain. A 10-minute brisk walk once a day is better than no exercise at all, and a 20-minute walk is even better. In other words, *any exercise is better than no exercise.*

The Ninety-Year-Old Man Who Wants to Die Running

Eventually, many people who acquire the exercise habit will want to begin jogging. It begins naturally when, instead of walking your entire exercise route, you jog for a short distance every so often. Many joggers started out by "jog-walking." However, you probably should not attempt to jog-walk until you can walk two or three 15-minute miles without getting tired.

What if you are fifty years old? Sixty? Seventy? Doesn't matter. You can get started on a personal exercise program, and you can benefit from it. In a television special on jogging, a 90-year-old jogger delighted viewers by showing his running form and by proclaiming the health-giving benefits of exercise. The interviewer asked the man if he thought he'd ever get too old to jog. "No," the man said with a grin. "I'm going to keep running as long as I can. I hope to die while I'm jogging." As fit as the man looked, he may live well beyond the century mark!

How You Can Exercise in Spite of Medical Problems

Medical problems, if they are not serious, shouldn't keep you from enjoying the benefits of exercise. In fact, walking regularly should work to your benefit. Among the medical conditions that improve with exercise are:

- *Diabetes.* Exercise helps the diabetic to lose weight. Also, exercise works to lower the blood sugar. Diabetics who take insulin usually find that they require less of it after they begin an exercise program.
- *Varicose veins.* Movement of the legs makes it easier for blood to flow through the veins. Losing weight by exercising is one of the best ways to heal varicose veins.
- *Poor circulation.* Some persons, usually men, develop

sluggish blood flow to the legs and feet. Walking causes pain in the legs, and the natural tendency is to stop until it goes away. Doctors used to treat this condition by telling the patient not to exercise. In recent years, though, it has become apparent that walking is the best treatment. Exercise stimulates the growth of new blood vessels and improves the circulation in general.

How Rudy M. Learned That Smoking
Does Have an Effect on the Heart

Rudy smoked. He was 55 and had smoked for 40 years. He had his first heart attack at the age of 50 and his second at the age of 54. Doctors at the hospital where Rudy was treated hit on a unique way of showing him why he should give up smoking. They injected a dye into his arm and then made x-ray pictures of his chest as the dye passed through his heart. The doctors had Rudy smoke a cigarette during a second dye injection. Later, they showed the patient the x-ray movies. Blood flowed normally to Rudy's heart during the first dye injection, but not the second. Every time Rudy took a puff on his cigarette, it caused his coronary arteries to shrink for a moment and carry less blood to his heart. This happened as long as he continued to inhale on the cigarette.

"You mean the blood supply to my heart shrinks up like that every time I take a puff on a cigarette?" Rudy asked.

"Yes," a doctor replied. "That's what smoking is doing to your heart."

Rudy didn't answer. He got up slowly and left the room. He didn't go around and announce that he was quitting, but quit he did. Within a week he was off of cigarettes for good—much to the benefit of his heart.

Protecting Yourself from This Silent Killer

Cigarette smoking is supposedly a pleasant habit, but it is also a killing one. A mild smoker is seven times as likely to die of lung cancer as a nonsmoker; a moderate smoker is twelve times as likely to die of lung cancer; and a heavy smoker is twenty-four times as likely to die of lung cancer as a nonsmoker. But cigarettes cause heart disease as well. Cigarette smokers have 70% more heart attacks than nonsmokers. *And the incidence of sudden death from heart attack is three times as great in smokers as in nonsmokers.*

The message is clear. If you smoke, stop. If you don't smoke, don't start.

Learning to Boost Your Heart Function by Conserving Your Energy

Sensible eating, exercise and not smoking can give you youth, health and longevity, but so can something else. That something is energy conservation. As a matter of fact, the heart does need its rest. It gets a time-out in between each heartbeat, and it beats slower and gets more rest when you exercise regularly. There is another way you can lessen its work: by losing weight if you are heavy. The fat person's heart must work harder even when the person is not moving around, and that's just the problem. Since the overweight individual doesn't get enough exercise, his heart is ill-equipped to stand the strain it is always under. There is hope! We'll see what can be done in the next chapter, *Staying Young by Losing Pounds the Natural Way.*

6

Staying Young by Losing Pounds the Natural Way

You can lose weight, and you can keep it off! However, to do so you will have to work at it, and the battle must continue even after those unsightly pounds have disappeared. The first step is to get rid of any false notions about how you gained weight in the first place.

How Joanna Learned the Truth about Weight Loss

Joanna was 50, weighed 220 pounds, and hadn't completely settled in her chair before she was telling me that she had been overweight since she was 18 years old and that she had a medical condition for her problem. "It's glandular. My thyroid gland is deficient."

Instead of answering Joanna right then, I proceeded with a thorough workup. On physical examination I found no evidence of thyroid disease. Except for her obesity, Joanna was in excellent health. "Well, of course the reason for that is that I'm on a thyroid hormone, doctor. I've been on it for several years, and it's really helped me."

"You've lost weight since you started taking it?"

"Well, no. I've stayed the same or gained a few pounds. But I feel better knowing I'm taking it."

The interesting thing to me as a doctor was that Joanna's dosage of thyroid was very, very small. She was taking only a fourth of a grain a day. If someone really needs thyroid medicine, they usually need at least two grains of it a day, or *eight times more than Joanna was taking*. I asked the patient to stop taking thyroid and then got some tests of her thyroid gland. All the tests were normal.

Confronted by the normal findings, Joanna grew red-faced with anger. "Well, if my thyroid is normal," she asked, "why am I overweight?"

Taking Advantage of Three Ways to Slim Down and Stay That Way

It was high time Joanna asked herself that question! The truth is, very few people are overweight because of a defective thyroid gland. One of the best doctors I've ever known has a large practice in a metropolitan area. He treats patients for heart disease, diabetes and other medical conditions, and also counsels people who want to lose weight. "How many of your overweight patients got that way because of a hormone imbalance or a thyroid problem?" I asked him. He snorted and said, "None! Overweight people with a glandular problem are rare as hen's teeth. And even if a patient has a glandular problem, he still gains weight the same way as anybody else!"

Joanna learned the truth about weight loss when she came to grips with the fact that she did not have a thyroid condition. She also learned and took advantage of the three ways to slim down and stay that way. These are:

(1) Eat fewer calories

(2) Increase your activity so that you will burn more calories

(3) Combine steps 1 and 2 for rapid weight loss

The Truth about Calories

The human body is a machine. To perform its work, it must have fuel in the form of food. What you eat is absorbed into your bloodstream and goes to cells throughout your body. The amount of energy yielded by a food depends on that food's content of carbohydrates, fats and proteins:

- *Carbohydrates yield 4 calories per gram of dry food weight.*
- *Proteins yield 4 calories per gram of dry food weight.*
- *Fats yield 9 calories per gram of dry food weight.*

In other words, fats give you *more than twice as many calories* as the same size helping of carbohydrate or protein. Sugar and potatoes are carbohydrates, and lean meat is protein. Butter, margarine and the fat from meat are fats, and eating such foods is the quickest way to get fat! Fat, after all, is stored energy. When you body can't use all the food that you eat, you get fat. All that stored energy ends up as unsightly, unhealthy, uncomfortable pounds of you know what! If fat is stored energy and the obese person has too much of it, why does he continue to get hungry and want to eat? I wish I knew. Nature made us the way we are, but then, nature didn't anticipate a society where food is abundant and inactivity so common that it is an accepted way of life. No matter. What's important to know is that if you are obese, you got that way by taking in more food calories than your body needed for energy. You can lose weight by going in the opposite direction. All you have to do is take in less food than your body burns for energy. It sounds simple, but there is a catch. *You—and no one else but you—must do the work and make the sacrifices necessary to lose weight.* The easy ways are never good, and the good ways are never easy.

Seven Tips You Can Use to Stay Young by Losing Pounds the Natural Way

A pound of fat is a storage vat containing 3,500 calories of energy. To lose this pound of fat you must burn up this 3,500 calories. In other words, you have to force your body to use its stores of fat for energy. One way to do this is to *eat fewer calories than your body needs.* Here are seven ways to do this:

#1. EAT ONLY WHEN YOU ARE HUNGRY.

Eating is a habit! If you're the kind of person who eats when you aren't really hungry, you may be able to lose weight simply by asking yourself one question before you put a bite of food into your mouth. The question is this : "What do I want most, this bite of food or the weight it's going to give me?"

**How Shelton N. Discovered
One Thing about Himself—
and Lost 50 Pounds**

Shelton, a 58-year-old postman, worked hard all day and liked to relax in the evenings. It was his life style, and he enjoyed it. What he didn't like was the fact that he had gained weight. He weighed 190 pounds, but wanted to weigh 140.

"I just don't eat that much," he told me, "and I know I get enough exercise carrying the mail. Yet the pounds just settle on my belly and won't come off."

His wife agreed. She was trim and healthy and said that she ate as much food as her husband. I asked Shelton what he did in the evenings *after* supper.

"Watch TV. We have a regular schedule of which programs to watch, and I glue myself to the set till bedtime."

"Ever snack while you watch?"

He grinned and nodded. "All the time."

It turned out that he had avocado dip at least once a week, though he also liked onion dip and bean dip. He dipped with corn chips or Doritos or Cheese Twists, and he washed his snacks down with a couple of cans of beer.

"But are you really hungry for the snacks? Is it eating that you truly desire because of an empty stomach, or is it eating out of habit?"

Shelton admitted that very often it was eating out of habit. I suggested that he eat a slightly larger supper and then not eat any snacks during the evening hours. On that plan alone, without going on a diet, Shelton lost 50 pounds. It took him two years to do it, but the good habits he learned during those two years will stay with him and help him keep the weight off for the rest of his life. I saw Shelton recently, and he said, "Doctor, if you want to tell people how they can lose weight, tell them to follow my rule. Don't ever, under any circumstances, eat while you're watching TV. Eating should take your full attention, and if you switch off that TV you're not going to eat unless you're hungry."

#2. SWITCH TO FRUIT FOR DESSERT.

Pudding, cake, doughnuts, candy—you name it. Rich desserts are loaded with fat, and this means that eating them makes you gain weight twice as fast as eating such things as lean meat or fruits. Give up pastries altogether and switch to fruits as your dessert. One cup of Tapioca cream pudding, for instance, contains 335 calories. Two doughnuts contain a total of 270 calories. By contrast, an apple supplies 70 calories, a banana about 85, half a grapefruit 55, an orange 65 and a peach 35. Switching to fruit for dessert can save you about 200 calories a day. A little less than three weeks of this will mean a weight loss of one pound. Not a lot of weight loss, and not rapidly, either. But added to the other pounds you are going to lose it can mean a slimmer, healthier you!

#3. SELECT LOW-CALORIE FOODS FOR SNACKS.

Eating while watching TV is not the only bad habit that has turned thin people into fat ones. Social eating, such as during a break or during a get-together, can mean the difference between losing weight and gaining it. The caution here is to beware of that "friend" who comes running at you with a cookie in one hand and a glass of punch in the other. The first thing you may have to learn is how to say no.

The Way George Avoided Eating Foods That He Didn't Need

I worked in the same building with George, but didn't see him too often. George was fat, and then one day someone told me he was sick. Not long after that I saw a man I thought was George, but I had trouble recognizing him. It was indeed George, but he had lost so much weight that he looked like a new man. My inquiry into his having been sick brought a grin to his face. He took me into his office and shut the door. "No, I haven't been sick," he said, "but I *have* been losing weight."

It had started with an attack of gallbladder trouble. George's doctor put him on a diet so he'd be ready in case surgery was necessary. But the people at the office were friendly, and almost every day one person or the other would bring cookies or cake or pie to work. "I didn't say a word about my diet, but people saw me losing weight, and you would have thought it was the worst thing I could do! Everyone wanted to feed me. So to keep from hurting their feelings I told them I wasn't feeling well and would rather not eat. And it worked; I've lost 70 pounds on this diet. But doctor, I had to tell the people I was sick, or they never would have let me reduce."

That his fellow workers didn't want to see George lose weight is unfortunate, but George's story is not all that uncommon. People don't offer you snacks to be mean, but out of a lack of understanding. In fact, most people you know would probably like to see you lose weight if you are overweight, but on the other hand it wouldn't bother them unduly to see you stay obese. By reducing, you create a change. Others have to adjust to the thin you and may unconsciously see you as a threat. Handle this with quiet determination. Stay away from office parties if at all possible and do select low-calorie foods for snacks.

Try keeping an assortment of carrots, celery and Melba toast on hand. One piece of Old London Wheat Melba Toast contains 16 calories, a carrot contains 20 calories, and a celery stalk (*without* pimento and cheese wedged into it) supplies 5 calories. For less than 50 calories, this trio can just about fill you up. Or, try a salad. Chopped and mixed, one carrot and half of a slice of pineapple make a refreshing salad that amounts to only 70 calories. By comparison, one average-sized cookie contains 70 or 75 calories, and how many people stop after eating only one cookie?

#4. SWITCH TO LOW-CAL DRINKS.

A twelve-ounce can of coke or other soft drink contains about 150 calories. Multiply this times two or three soft drinks a day, and in a couple of weeks you've got an extra 3,500 calories—the equivalent of a pound of fat! Too many people forget that a can of beer provides 150 calories, and one drink of whiskey, gin or vodka will supply about 75-100 calories. The best idea is to switch to low-calorie drinks.

Many persons enjoy the natural taste of tea or coffee—without adding sugar. At the most, unsweetened tea or coffee will give you only 2 or 3 calories a serving. Limit your coffee intake to no more than four cups a day, but you can drink up to six glasses or cups of tea before noticing any side effects such as slight nervousness or a mild increase in heart rate.

Club soda with a twist of lemon or a dash of lime can be delicious, and it contains no calories. Or, squeeze half a cup of grapefruit juice, add water or club soda, and drink it over crushed ice. (Top it with a strawberry.) This drink contains only 40 to 50 calories. A similar concoction can be made using orange juice or apple juice, but the calorie content will be slightly higher. Use your ingenuity to think of other low-cal drinks.

#5. LEARN TO USE AS LITTLE SUGAR AS POSSIBLE.

Eating sugar adds calories to your diet, and may harm your heart and other organs. For better health—and a thinner body— learn to use as little sugar as possible. Don't eat presweetened cereal and sugary desserts. Cut down on the amount of sugar you add to recipes. Drink your coffee or tea straight, or with a bit of low-fat milk. Don't be surprised to discover that the natural taste of a food or drink is better than the syrupy-sweet taste you thought you liked. And if you must have something sweet, make it honey instead of sugar.

#6. MAKE THAT EVENING OUT A MOVIE NOT A MEAL.

Eating out is fun! That's because the food is plentiful and you don't have to prepare it. But the pleasure of having a good time tends to strain your willpower to the breaking point. You overeat. *Don't eat out if you're trying to lose weight!* If you need a night out, go to a movie or a play. It's better not to go to someone's house for dinner, either, because that can be worse than dining out in a restaurant. The choice for someone with an active social life is very difficult, and also very simple. The choice is: "Do I lose weight, or don't I?"

The Way Helen Used Her Talents
to Lose Weight Instead of Gaining It

She weighed an even 200 pounds, and much of it had been gained at fund-raising banquets or brunches or other social events. Helen was a lovely woman, and she was very active in her community. "What am I going to do about my social life?" she asked when it became clear that she would not be able to continue eating the way she was eating and still lose the 75 pounds she wanted to lose.

I pointed out that if she could devote even half the energy to doing something about her overweight as she did to bettering the community, she'd have no trouble trimming down. She went one better than that. She channeled her activities into forming a weight-reducing club in her city; the last I heard it was still going strong, and as its leader and main beneficiary Helen was helping to spread the good word to other people. She was also wearing a size 12 dress for the first time in ten years.

#7. CHOOSE A SENSIBLE DIET THAT INCLUDES ALL CLASSES OF FOODS.

The grapefruit diet, the honey diet, the drinking man's diet, the quick-weight-loss diets—you've probably heard of these and many others. They're gimmicks! They promise you something, and many times you do lose weight on the diet, but what then? The point is that STAYING THIN is as important as losing the weight in the first place. Therefore, why go on some exotic diet? Your goal should be to lose a pound or a pound and a half a week, and you can do this by following the advice in this chapter. Create your own "diet" from the same foods others in your family are eating. How much you eat is more important than what you eat, though you should try to follow the rules for sensible eating and cooking given in the previous chapter, and you should follow the low-salt suggestions given in Chapter 4.

The diet below supplies about 1,500 to 1,600 calories a day. It includes breakfast, a mid-morning snack, lunch, a mid-afternoon snack, dinner and a bedtime snack. You might wish to eat only three times a day, and if so, you could eat an extra helping of food at two of the three meals. Just keep in mind that you should enjoy good nutrition while you diet. In fact, eating a variety of foods is probably going to give you a more contented, comfortable feeling than going on a fad diet that sooner or later must come to an end.

The Six-Feedings Diet (1,500-1,600 calories)

BREAKFAST

> Coffee or tea—no sugar added; or, an eight-ounce glass of low-fat milk.
> One piece of toast with one teaspoon of jelly
> Fruit juice (optional)

MID-MORNING SNACK

> One cup of tea or coffee—no sugar added
> One or two pieces of Melba toast (optional)

LUNCH

One sandwich on whole wheat or whole rye bread, with tomatoes, lettuce, low-cal mayonnaise, and two or three thin slices of pressed chicken or pressed beef
One apple, orange or peach; or, half a grapefruit
One cup of tea or coffee—no sugar added

MID-AFTERNOON SNACK

One chopped carrot, sweetened with half a slice of pineapple
Or, two pieces of Melba toast

DINNER

One meat
Two vegetables
Small salad (low-cal dressing)
One piece of whole wheat or whole rye bread
Coffee or tea, unsweetened

BEFORE-BEDTIME SNACK

One piece of fruit, or two pieces of Melba toast

Vanessa's Discovery of Calorie Burning and How She Used It to Lose Fifteen Pounds

Like most people, Vanessa had heard all of her life about how to lose weight: you go on a diet. "The trouble with me," she said with dejection, "is that I start watching what I eat, lose a few pounds, and then the first thing I know I'm right back up there again. I just wish someone would invent a way to make it easier to take those pounds off and keep them off."

Happily, I had an answer for Vanessa: calorie burning. I told her about a study that had appeared in the prestigious *Journal of the American Medical Association.* "They've proven that you can lose weight by exercising regularly and not going on a diet. The study was done in California. A group of overweight women was weighed and told to walk briskly for 30 minutes or more a day. The ladies didn't go on a diet, and some of them actually began to eat more than they had before the exercise program. Yet at the end of a year on the program, each woman had lost an average of 22 pounds."

Exercise does burn calories, and Vanessa began her own program of walking and riding a bicycle. As of this writing she hasn't been on the program quite a year, but she has lost fifteen pounds. "The nicest thing about exercising is that I can eat a little more if I want to and not gain weight. And if I cut down on my eating and exercise, too, the weight just melts off!"

The Way to Eat and Still Lose Weight

Vanessa's discovery was new to her, but people have been enjoying the weight-losing benefits of exercise for many, many years. Using your body burns calories and helps to melt away that energy you've stored in the form of fat. Most kids are slim, despite eating enormous amounts of food. Kids stay slim because of their activities. They don't walk, they run. They play ball, ride bicycles, swim, bowl, knock around up and down the street, or just take off running for the sheer joy of running. Activity is the secret of youth, and you can cash in on this secret by exercising. Here are the numbers of calories you can burn during various activities:

Type of exercise	Calories burned per hour
Walking	300
Jogging	600
Bicycling	400
Swimming	500
Tennis	400
Bowling	270
Golf (no cart or caddy)	300
Dancing	330

Now let's put these activities to use for you. In the last chapter I recommended you walk an hour a day to keep your heart and vessels young. Doing so, you'll burn 300 calories a day over and above the calories you use during your ordinary activities. Let's do some calculating. Multiply 300 calories a day times seven days in a week, and you have a total of 2,100 calories burned during that week. Two weeks would mean 4,200 calories—over a pound of weight loss. In a year's time, walking an hour a day will take off 30 pounds. Doesn't sound like much? Then let me ask you a question. Do you weigh 30 pounds less than you weighed a year ago? A year from now the answer could be yes—if you begin a program of walking an hour a day. You'll invigorate your heart and vessels, too.

It's all right to vary the exercise program. Too cold to walk outdoors? Go bowling! Shop in an enclosed mall and make some extra trips up and down the length of it. Or get an exercycle. The important thing is that you get started moving around and burning calories. And remember, to get the most out of calorie burning, the exercise has to be over and above your ordinary activities.

Try This Twenty-Minute Refresher

Don't have an hour to exercise? Then walk briskly for 20 minutes each day. Here's how to turn even this relatively small amount of time into a weight-losing program:

- *Spend a minute or two doing the hamstring and calf-stretching exercises described in Chapter 4.*
- *Note the time and stride off briskly. Walk in one direction for ten minutes.*
- *At the end of ten minutes, turn around and walk back to your starting point.*

The twenty minutes of walking will burn about 100 calories. In a week's time this will add up to 700 calories. Five weeks of the 20-minute-a-day program will add up to 3,500 calories. This means that in a year you can lose over 10 pounds just by walking for 20 minutes each day! (Assuming, of course, that you do not increase your food intake.) More than helping you to lose weight, the 20 minutes of exercise will make you feel better. That is why I call it a 20-minute refresher. It's like charging your batteries: It benefits brain, body and vessels. And you can take advantage of it during your lunch hour if that's the only spare time you have during the day.

The Secret of Youth Is as Near as the Street

Exercise can help you lose weight, and it can keep you young. As you grow older, your bulk tends to shift; you lose muscle at the expense of gaining fat. Weight leaves the shoulders and chest and accumulates in the tummy and hips. Your trunk gets bigger and your legs get smaller. It's a frustrating experience, but exercise, by keeping the muscles trim, tends to reverse these changes or keep them from occurring. That's why moving about and using your body comes as close as anything to being the secret of youth.

How Norman Learned to Set
Realistic Goals—and Achieve Them

Norman was a 40-year-old man who weighed 280 pounds. His problem wasn't that he wouldn't diet, but that he set his goals too high. He'd try to lose 50 pounds in a month, and fail. Whereupon he'd go on an eating binge that would make him fatter than when he started. He grew very discouraged. "Doc," he told me, "I'd give anything to get back down to the two-twenty I weighed two years ago. I'm eating myself to death. I not only don't lose, I keep right on gaining. I wish I could just figure out some way to hold my own."

"That sounds like a pretty good goal," I said. "Let's set up a reward program for you. Buy some gold stars and a sheet of poster board. Weigh yourself every week, and for a week when you don't gain, put three gold stars beside your name on the poster board. And if you lose weight that week, put six gold stars out there. We'll see how many stars you can earn in a month."

Norman loved it! He called each week to share his results with me, and at the end of a month he had earned 18 gold stars. He was proud that he had learned to hold his own and even lose some weight, and he'd realized something. "Doc, it's better to set a small goal and achieve it than to shoot for the moon and fail. My confidence is up, and I'm going to stick with this."

In a year's time Norman was able to lose 30 pounds. He is still very obese, but he is reducing. With each pound he loses he gains confidence in his ability to shed weight and keep it off.

How to Be Your Own Best Friend

We all work for rewards, but losing weight is its own best reward. Looking slim and getting more fun out of life are the "gold stars" you earn by losing weight. Set a realistic goal for yourself and achieve it. And as you lose weight, learn to enjoy the new you that appears in the mirror. Primp! Do your hair differently! Buy new clothes. Think of yourself as thin, act thin, and above all, stay that way.

How do you stay thin?

By being your own best friend.

Which means combining diet and exercise to stay slim. You can do it, but you are the *only one* who can do it for *you*. And by keeping those unwanted pounds from sneaking back, you really are being your own best friend.

7

Making Use of Home Treatments
to Relieve the Pain and Stiffness
of Arthritis

Pain and stiffness are only two of the symptoms of arthritis. Your arthritis may interfere with your daily activities, or it may cause your hands and knees to swell. Your back and neck may be so stiff each morning that you have to unlimber before you can begin the day's activities. Or your problem may be somewhat different. No matter. There is much that you can do to relieve these symptoms. And the nice thing is that you can choose from common materials available in your own home.

Choosing One of Five Methods to Treat Arthritis

You can choose from the following five methods to get relief from arthritis:

1. *Apply heat to the painful joints.*
2. *Do range of motion exercises.*
3. *Get plenty of rest.*
4. *Put gravity to work for you.*
5. *Use the one drug that helps the most.*

Actually, the best way to get relief from your arthritis is to use a combination of these five methods. Heat provides quick relief from pain, and range of motion exercises and rest are measures that will cut down on pain and stiffness. Taking a drug to get relief from pain can be reserved for when other measures don't work. Too many arthritis patients make the mistake of assuming that drugs are the *only* treatment. When the drug fails to relieve the pain, the sufferer becomes discouraged and asks for a stronger medicine. This would not happen nearly so often if the person would first turn to such soothing, satisfying measures as heat, exercise and rest.

How Sally D. Caught On to a Little-Known Way to Treat Arthritis

Sally D., a victim of osteoarthritis, or "bony arthritis," was a retired school teacher who thought that she had seen everything. Young at 58, she loved to participate in various social clubs and organizations. Flowers were her main love, but she did not neglect birdwatching, reading and home canning. One year she was having a particularly hard time with arthritis in her fingers, and she noticed something during the process of putting up some peach preserves. The paraffin for the seal on the bottles got on her hands, and it was like, in her words, "I had just been given a hand transplant. I began to move my fingers better, the pain was gone, and I felt great!" Sally spent a marvelous afternoon in the kitchen and called her doctor to say that she had gotten relief from the warm paraffin. "Why don't they tell people this is a good treatment for arthritis?" she asked.

Her physician told her that paraffin was already a well-recognized treatment for the relief of arthritis pain, but that it was used mainly in the hospital. And the benefit comes not from the paraffin itself, but from the heat used to melt it. The paraffin holds the heat and releases it slowly and soothingly to the patient's hands.

Five Ways to Use Heat to Relieve Pain and Stiffness

Heat to an arthritic joint is like salve to a sunburn: blessed relief! By warming tissues, heat increases blood flow. Relief of pain occurs because joint motion is made easier. Here are five ways to take advantage of either *dry heat* or *moist heat*:

(1) The heat lamp. A heat lamp provides dry heat. You can use an ordinary goosenecked desk lamp with a 100-watt bulb or purchase a special heat lamp from a medical supply store. A heat lamp with a 250-watt Mazda CX bulb can be plugged into an ordinary electrical outlet, but be sure to read the instructions before using this or any other heating light. For example, it's a good idea to put something between the lamp and your skin to protect yourself from the glare. A towel, folded once or twice, is perfectly adequate. Keep the light source at least 18 to 24 inches from your skin.

At first, use heat treatments only a few minutes a day and then gradually work up to the point of treating your troublesome joints for ten minutes three times a day. Much of the pain and stiffness of arthritis comes from the muscles around the joint. Heat brings gentle relief. Remember that you can defeat the pain-relieving effects of heat if you apply it for too long at one time. Overexposure to a hot light can cause your skin and muscles to ache.

(2) The heating pad. The heating pad also provides dry heat, and its advantages are obvious. It is more convenient than using a heat lamp, because you can wrap it around a painful knee to treat the entire joint. A bonus of using a heating pad is that you don't have to worry as much about overheating your skin, though it is possible for this to occur.

Electric heating pads can be bought in many stores. They are available in department stores and at medical supply stores. You can turn an electric blanket into an excellent heating pad, and on a chilly day drawing the entire blanket around you may be a good way to relieve morning stiffness.

Begin therapy with a heating pad slowly, and work up to using it several times a day, usually for no more than ten minutes at a time. Take the pad with you when you go on a trip, and use it anywhere that electricity is available.

(3) Hot bath. Hot water gives off moist heat, of course, and a tub full of piping hot water provides about the quickest and certainly the most relaxing form of heat therapy that you can enjoy.

Run the bath water high enough so that you can get everything but your face and head under water, and plan to keep the water temperature at about 100° F. This temperature is hotter than you might imagine, so you may have to start out with the water a little cooler. Soak in the hot water for 20 or 30 minutes, draining water and adding more hot water to keep the temperature near its original level. You may use heat in the form of a hot bath once or twice a day.

(4) Blankets or towels dipped in hot water. Some persons are unable to get into a tub. With proper help, such people can still experience the pleasure of a hot tub bath. Have an assistant place a rubber sheet on your bed to protect the mattress from water. Place an old blanket on top of the rubber sheet, and then climb on top of this blanket. The assistant, having folded it lengthwise for quick unfolding, dips a cotton sheet into a tub of hot water. Then he folds this piping hot sheet under and around you. The final step is to wrap the blanket around your body to hold in the heat. If the room is warm the heat should last for 15 or 20 minutes.

A face towel or a wash rag can be dipped into a basin of hot water and used to apply moist heat to your joints. This is a convenient way to apply heat to only one or two joints. Dip the cloth into the hot water as often as you wish, and treat your painful joints for 10 or 15 minutes.

(5) Warm paraffin bath. Paraffin holds heat and seems to help it penetrate into the skin. The paraffin bath is generally used to help the person with rheumatoid arthritis, but it can benefit the patient with bony arthritis of the fingers. You can purchase a home paraffin unit to heat the waxy material. Melt four pounds of paraffin and several ounces of mineral oil or petrolatum jelly in a double boiler. Let the mixture of paraffin and mineral oil cool until a thin white coating appears on top, and then dip your hands (or feet) into the mixture several times until a glove (sock) of paraffin covers them. You may want to let the paraffin cover your painful wrists or ankles, too. Take care not to move your fingers or toes during the coating. Afterward, wrap the paraffin-covered areas with wax paper and a towel, and relax for 15 or 20 minutes.

When the paraffin has cooled, you can peel it from your hands and return it to the container for reuse. Use paraffin heat treatments three times a day for symptomatic relief when your hands are hurting.

The Benefits You Can Expect

How much relief you get from heat will depend on the severity and location of your arthritis. Some people get more relief than others. As one patient told me, "Doctor, I wouldn't leave home without my heat blanket, especially in the cold months. I used to wonder why my arthritis bothered me more in the cold weather, and I guess it was because of the stiffness. Using heat gives me back my hands, and I'll never go without it." The best results come from using heat along with other methods of treatment.

How Maxine Z. Learned to Keep
Her Hands and Shoulders
Free from Stiffness

Maxine was different. She was young, attractive and a concert pianist. She had everything to look forward to, but then it happened. The orchestra with which she was touring swung into the South, and one rainy morning in Louisiana Maxine woke up with stiff fingers. It frightened her so badly she stayed all day in her room, refusing to perform that evening. Next morning she had pain as well as stiffness in her fingers. By then, Maxine was frantic. She had known all along that her mother was a victim of bony arthritis, and now Maxine had to face the fact that she, too, might have osteoarthritis. She visited a physician, who did some tests and told her to come back in two weeks. At the return visit the doctor confirmed the diagnosis of early arthritis and prescribed some medicine to relieve the symptoms. The medicine didn't work. In the following months Maxine's pain and stiffness got worse, and it spread to her elbows and shoulders. She lost the coordination in her hands and had to resign her seat in the orchestra. Returning to New York, Maxine gave up all hopes of continuing her career. What she hadn't counted on was her mother's insistence that she see the same specialist who had been treating her for several years. At the very first visit, Maxine made a discovery.

THE DISCOVERY OF RANGE OF MOTION EXERCISES

"Maxine," the specialist told her, "lots of people have arthritis, and have it even worse than you. Yet they can still go on about their activities, and yes, even play the piano. In fact, there's a way you can treat your stiffness that probably hasn't occurred to you. You're a pianist, did you ever do those finger exercises they do?"

"Certainly. But exercising is impossible now that my arthritis has gotten so bad."

"But that's just the point. To get the best possible use out of your fingers, exercise is more important than ever. You need to start moving your fingers every day. Here's what I want you to do."

THE ADVANTAGE OF EXERCISING REGULARLY

The rheumatologist (a specialist in the care of arthritis) told Maxine to go through range of motion exercises three times a day. He stressed that to derive maximum benefit from them, Maxine had to do the exercises regularly.

Because the first few sessions were painful, Maxine learned to use a heat pad for 15 minutes immediately before putting her fingers and shoulders through their normal ranges of motion. The heat treatment made the unlimbering easier, and she was soon able to flex and extend and wiggle her fingers for 10 minutes three times a day. Maxine Z. did eventually begin to play the piano again, and though she did not rejoin the same orchestra, she was able to once again perform in public. But even today, she continues doing her range of motion exercises several times a day.

Getting Full Movement in Spite of Arthritis

A joint is the space, or hinge, between two bones. Joints make movement possible, and each joint has a normal range of motion, a certain distance that you can comfortably move it. Arthritis, by causing pain in the joint, keeps you from moving it so well. The natural tendency is to rest the part that hurts, but this is exactly the wrong thing to do. Unless you continue to exercise an arthritic joint, it will just get stiffer and stiffer. Eventually, you could lose almost all of its motion. Range of motion exercises keep your arthritic joints working to their fullest extent. It is always easier to prevent a loss of motion than to correct it after it has occurred, but exercise will help you move even the stiffest of joints.

The Exercises to Perform

Since stiffness is worst first thing in the morning, start each day with range of motion exercises. Then, repeat the movements at midday and again before retiring that night. Select from the following exercises according to where you have arthritis:

- *Shoulders.* Ordinarily, you should be able to extend your arms straight up, straight forward, straight down and about 45° backward. Carry the arms through these motions several times.

- *Wrists.* You can sway your wrists slightly to either side of the midline and bend and raise them. A normal wrist should bend to at least a 90° angle with the forearm, and you should be able to pull it backward to well above the normal line of the forearm. Move your wrists through these motions three times a day.

- *Elbows.* You should be able to straighten your forearm out from your body or bend it until it touches your upper arm. Again, do these range of motion exercises three times daily and work up to the full range of motion slowly.

- *Fingers and hands.* Straighten each finger and then curl it up. Concentrate on doing this several times per finger and then for all the fingers at once. You can do both hands at the same time. Exercise your hand by balling your fist, straightening the hand, and balling it again.

- *Knees.* Lie with your back on the floor. Straighten one leg completely, and then bend it as much as possible. A normal knee will bend enough to let your heel touch your buttock. Repeat the motion five times for each leg. Do not force the movement, because you'll find that it gets easier to do week by week.

- *Upper spine.* Sit in a comfortable chair and move your

head back and forth so that at one extreme your chin touches your chest, and at the other extreme the back of your head reaches your spine. Let your head fall to one side and then the other. Repeat these movements of your head five times each.

- *Lower spine.* Stand with your hands on your hips. Bend forward from the waist and then straighten your spine and push your tummy out. Repeat this exercise five times. Hands still on your hips, lean first to one side and then to the other for five times each. To strengthen your lower back muscles, lie on your back. Tense your buttocks and raise your lower spine off the floor. Relax and let your spine return to the starting position. Repeat the exercise five times.

What Exercise Will Do for You

Range of motion exercises may be painful if you aren't used to them. However, the first limbering up is the most difficult. If you feel uncomfortable after the exercising, you're doing too much too fast. Continue to exercise, but at a slower rate. Also, if exercise causes swelling in a joint, go easy.

During the exercise you may hear some creaking in your joints if you have osteoarthritis. These creaking or crunching sounds occur for several reasons. Some joint creaking is normal and occurs even in persons who don't have arthritis. Calcium grows in and around the joints of people who have arthritis, and these mineral deposits can bind against one another during motion of the joint. Creaking of your joints will not be a problem if you perform the exercises slowly, working to widen the range of movement a little at a time. You may eventually want to repeat each exercise more than five times.

After you've exercised your joints for a few days or weeks, you'll note freer motion. You'll begin to reach for things and not experience the twinge of pain you used to feel. By increasing the joint's range of motion, you will have eased yourself of a great deal of pain. A point that is worth repeating is that heat therapy and exercise go hand in hand. Some people prefer to use heat first and follow it with range of motion exercises, while others prefer to unlimber and then use heat. Do what works best for you.

Importance of Body Movement

Range of motion exercises should not be your only activity. You need a good exercise program. Swimming is especially good exercise for the person with arthritis of the hips or knees. However, walking can help just as much, so long as the walk doesn't take you into the bitter cold. One other thing the victim of arthritis needs is plenty of rest.

Giving Your Body What It Needs

One of the most unusual cases of osteoarthritis on record occurred in a 46-year-old woman quite suddenly one winter. This lady, in addition to caring for her own family and holding a part-time job, was thrust into a political campaign that taxed her energies. Two weeks before the election her mother had a stroke, further draining the daughter's energies. The election arrived; her candidate won. But the woman was too bushed to take any pleasure out of the victory. In fact, she could not get out of bed the next morning. She noted some stiffness in her joints and a slight fever, and doctors eventually diagnosed the condition as arthritis. The drain of the political campaign and her mother's illness had weakened this woman's resistance. Doctors don't always understand how such things happen, but they do recognize that arthritis often begins during a time of considerable fatigue.

This particular lady, Louise Ann B., was told that she had to give up her job, had to give up politics, and had to limit her wide-ranging activities. "But if I don't do these things, who will?" she asked.

"You may eventually be able to get back to them," the doctor replied, "but first things first. Right now you have to get your arthritis under control. You're run-down, you're underweight, you're weak and you've got arthritis in your fingers, wrists and elbows. I want you to stay in bed for a week until you begin to get your strength back, and then you're going to have to continue to take it easy."

The physician was right in putting Louise Ann to bed for a week, because she did feel much better when her strength returned. By organizing her time, she was able to do most of the things she wanted to do. But one mistake she made no more was to let herself get too tired. Rest, Louise Ann learned, is a very important part of arthritis therapy.

Choosing What Works Best for You

How much rest you need depends on your age, health, activities, and the severity of your symptoms. Here are some guidelines:

• *Rest when you feel tired.* We all get tired, even those of us who do not have arthritis. But fatigue is actually one of the symptoms of arthritis, and it is a warning that you need to rest. Tiredness comes from the muscles around the painful joint. These muscles are under a strain. They must work harder when a joint is out of line, and yet they can't pull as well because of the friction of calcium deposits near the joint. The best way to relieve the tiredness is to rest.

• *Take an afternoon rest.* Most patients find it convenient to lie down for about an hour in the afternoon. A siesta can be most refreshing, because it will give your muscles the rest they need for the remainder of the day's activities!

• *Keep regular hours.* Get into the habit of going to sleep at a certain time of the day and continue this excellent habit. If you know that you must get up by a certain time, go to bed early enough that you'll wake up before the alarm goes off. Why? For a good reason: *If you're getting all the sleep you need, you should wake up on your own!* Another benefit of waking up before the alarm goes off is that you'll have time to do your morning exercises before starting the day's activities.

• *Keep what you do within tolerable limits.* A man came to see me because of arthritis in his knee. Years before, John W. had injured the knee playing football, but the pain had gotten so bad lately that it was giving him fits. "It's worse on Monday," he said. "I call it my Monday arthritis. If I could get through the first part of the week without having to limp around, I'd have it made."

"John," I said, "maybe we ought to talk about what you do on Sunday. Anything out of the ordinary?"

He thought about it. "Read the morning paper. Church. Lunch. Maybe watch TV. Oh, there is one thing. Lately I've been getting into a pretty good game of football with my kids and some of the neighborhood children. But that's nothing. You don't think that could be causing my Monday arthritis, do you? Come to think of it, doc, I don't believe I was having this much trouble on Monday until we started having those Sunday football games."

The man had answered my question and solved his problem at the same time. An awareness of what he was doing wrong was all he needed, and he stopped having "Monday arthritis" when he stopped playing Sunday football.

Do not stop your activities, because that would be giving in to the arthritis. But do keep strenuous tasks at a reasonable level. This means you shouldn't attempt to do the things that you cannot tolerate. As for weekend sports activities, the rule is this: You don't play games to get your arthritis into shape. You get your arthritis into shape so that you will be able, perhaps, to play games.

• *Combination of exercise and rest is best.* Just because you need rest does not mean that you can't exercise your joints and also get involved in a regular form of exercise yourself, such as swimming or walking. A good program would be to do the range of motion exercises first thing in the morning and again at noon and bedtime. Your daily walk or swim would fit best in the early afternoon, just before or after your daily rest period.

Six Ways to Take Advantage of Gravity

The pull of the earth's gravity affects everything that we do. Simply walking upright goes against gravity, and if your posture is bad the pull of gravity on your spine is going to be uneven. The following six suggestions will help you to turn gravity to your advantage in getting relief from arthritis:

(1) *Keep your weight evenly distributed.* When walking or standing, keep your weight as evenly distributed as possible. In other words, try not to give in or favor an arthritic knee or hip. The added pressure you put on the "good" leg will hasten its tendency to develop arthritis. Try to avoid walking stiff-legged or flat-footed.

(2) *Walk with your head up, chin in and shoulders back.* This

keeps your spine in the best possible alignment and balances the gravitational pull on your torso.

(3) Try to get by without a cane. If you must use a cane, do. However, a cane is a way of favoring one leg or the other, and it is better to keep your weight evenly distributed on both legs.

(4) Learn to sit properly. Sit in a firm chair with both feet on the floor and your hips and shoulders against the back of the chair. This keeps your spine in the best possible alignment, while providing the needed support for your legs and shoulders.

(5) Sleep on a firm bed. Make sure your bed is firm enough to adequately support your body weight. Purchase the firmest "orthopedic" mattress you can find. Or, you can support your present mattress by inserting a piece of ⅜-inch plyboard between it and the boxsprings. Cut the plyboard so that it is about two feet wide and four or five feet long.

(6) Use one small pillow. Sleep on a small pillow, one only, since large pillows force you to sleep with your spine bent. Don't use pillows to prop up your knees, since sleeping with your legs bent encourages them to be stiff and painful the next morning.

Using the One Drug That Helps the Most

The drug that is most helpful to the arthritic person is *aspirin*. The "arthritis pain formulas" you see advertised on television contain aspirin as the basic ingredient. The ones that are supposedly stronger than aspirin because of the presence of extra ingredients are not really that much stronger, and some of these ingredients can be harmful to you.

How Merrill Learned
the Truth about Pain Relievers

Merrill P. had osteoarthritis and was bothered by pain during his work on an automobile assembly line. For years he had gotten by without drugs, but he kept hearing them advertised on television. One weekend he purchased a "pain formula" containing aspirin and phenacetin and began to take it several times a day. His pains lessened, and then he developed another problem. He began having to get up several times during the night to make urine. He had a dull ache in his back and flank. A physician ran some tests and discovered that Merrill's kidneys weren't functioning properly. As soon as the doctor learned that Merrill had been taking large doses of phenacetin, he made a tentative diagnosis of *renal papillary necrosis.* This kidney condition used to be quite rare, but starting in the early 1950's doctors began to see a lot of patients with it. Almost every such person had been taking large doses of pain formulas containing phenacetin. The real tragedy was that these people could have gotten just as much relief from taking aspirin alone!

Merrill? He was fortunate. The disease was not advanced, and when he stopped poisoning himself with phenacetin, his kidneys recovered. Now Merrill takes aspirin when he takes something for his arthritis. He takes aspirin and nothing else, *unless the medicine is prescribed by a physician.*

Here are some tips on the use of aspirin:

• *One form of aspirin is as good as another!* The so-called "name brands" of aspirin usually cost more than the other brands. During a recent comparison of prices, I found that I could purchase 500 "off brand" aspirin tablets for less than what it would have cost to buy 200 "name brand" aspirin tablets. As a physician, I know that government regulations require all makers of aspirin to use care and skill in its preparation. Also, the drug itself, acetylsalicylic acid, is the same no matter what brand name is stamped on the bottle's label. It makes sense to *purchase the least expensive brand of aspirin you can find.* Supermarkets and discount stores sell inexpensive brands of aspirin.

• *Take aspirin for relief of pain.* A patient told me, "I don't know why I got that pain in my hands while I was playing tennis. I took two aspirin before I went out on the court." What this woman did not realize was that aspirin doesn't work very well in preventing pain. It works quite well in giving you relief from pain that is already present. Reserve aspirin for the pain that does not go away despite heat and other treatments, and remember this:

Aspirin helps to relieve the pain of arthritis, but it does not improve arthritis or cure it.

   • *Aspirin should be used as a drug.* The standard aspirin tablet contains 300 mg. of aspirin. The usual dose is two such tablets every three or four hours for relief of pain. Like any drug, aspirin has certain side effects. It can irritate the lining of your stomach and intestine, and it can cause ringing in your ears when you take too much of it. Some people get nauseated after taking aspirin; persons who suffer from an ulcer of the stomach can experience bleeding from the ulcer after taking aspirin. Here are three important rules:

1. *Take no more than eight aspirin tablets a day.* This means you can take two tablets on four separate occasions during the day. If you feel that you need more aspirin than this, check with your physician. The doctor can prescribe a longer-acting form of aspirin, such as sodium or potassium salicylate, and these compounds can be taken in slightly higher doses than regular aspirin.

2. *Wash the aspirin down with water or low-fat milk.* You will do your stomach and intestines a favor if you wash aspirin down with a glass of water or milk. The liquid helps to dilute the medicine for rapid absorption and also protects the lining of the stomach. If possible, it's a good idea to take aspirin at mealtime. That way, the food itself guards the stomach lining.

3. *Be cautious about taking aspirin when you have stomach problems.* Because the drug can irritate the stomach, you should not take it if you have a history of stomach ulcer, gastritis or a similar problem. You run the risk of worsening the ulcer or even causing it to bleed. A physician is the best person to advise you on what pain relievers you can safely take when you have an ulcer or intestinal problems.

Two Things That Can Make
All the Difference in Your
Winning Fight against Arthritis

I have saved the most important points for last. There are two of them, and if you can succeed at these two things you shouldn't have any trouble accomplishing the rest of the program discussed in this chapter. The two most important things in your winning fight against arthritis are:

(1) Losing weight if you are overweight

(2) Learning not to give in to the disease

Weight loss is the subject of Chapter 6, and losing weight if you are obese is probably the single most important thing you can do to make your arthritis better. Your bones and the joints between those bones must support your weight as you move around. Being overweight taxes the joints and hastens the destructive processes of arthritis. Almost everyone over the age of 30 has a little bit of osteoarthritis. However, the frequency of this condition in obese persons leaves no doubt that the more weight the bones must support, the greater the chances for arthritis to occur. To repeat, losing weight is the most pain-relieving thing that you can do.

The Decision That Changed Ramona's Life

Ramona was a 50-year-old member of the Hospital Auxiliary. She helped out in Arthritis Clinic, and I came to rely on her to fill out laboratory slips, to show patients the way to the pharmacy, or to do a dozen other things. The person with arthritis can become discouraged, and Ramona was especially adept at showing with a smile and a friendly word of encouragement that things would get better, that things would be okay.

One day I got a shock. Ramona and I were helping an elderly man into a wheelchair when I happened to notice that her hands were as gnarled and twisted as the roots of an old tree.

"You have arthritis," I said. "I didn't know."

"Had it ten years, doctor, the worst kind of arthritis. It's why I like to work here, and why I love to encourage the people that things *will* get better. Why, I was one of the most pitiful women you ever saw when I first got it. I cried and withdrew and told myself I'd rather be dead. Then one day my 16-year-old daughter read me something from a book she brought home from school. I'm sure you've heard it. It went, 'I had no shoes, and I murmured—until I met a man who had no feet.' Right then I made my decision. I could either give in to the arthritis or fight it. I chose to fight. I got up out of a chair in the back room and went into the kitchen and started making dinner for my family. It was the first time I'd fixed a meal in months. And it hurt to move, believe me. But it's gotten easier and easier every day since then."

Like Ramona, you must make the decision to fight back. Here are the three ways you can do this:

(1) Continue your life in spite of arthritis. Don't think of yourself as a cripple. Think of yourself as you. Look upon arthritis as a temporary inconvenience. At worst it is a detour, not a roadblock. In spite of the pain and misery of arthritis, the disease does not shorten your life span. You can live with it, and you can live in spite of it!

(2) Find your relief in healthy living. Exercise, rest, weight reduction and the timely use of aspirin will bring relief from the pain and stiffness of arthritis. Don't be taken in by an advertisement for a "cure," because all such claims are quackery. Healthy living and the program outlined in this chapter are all you need to get relief from arthritis.

(3) Take an active part in your own care. Doctors are busy people, and yours may not have told you about using heat, range of motion exercises and other things to relieve your symptoms. Learning to treat yourself will make you an expert in arthritis therapy and assure you of always having "expert" care. What is more, you may be able to slow the progress of the disease and greatly reduce your symptoms. The goal is well worth the effort required to reach it!

8

Keeping Your Kidneys Fit by Using the Least Expensive Medicine in the World

The kidneys are filters. Two-hundred quarts of fluid a day pour through them, and all but a quart of it is returned to the bloodstream. That one quart, expelled as urine, flushes out the chemical waste products from your bloodstream. The kidneys are tremendous organs, and one thing that makes them so tremendous is that you can use the least expensive medicine in the world to keep them healthy and young.

How Etta B. Learned That the Least Expensive Medicines Are Often the Best

Etta B. had a problem with her urine, but she was unwilling to explain the details of the problem over the phone. Instead, she insisted I meet her at the emergency room of a local hospital. As I drove to the hospital I tried to imagine what was wrong. Etta was about 50, worked as a receptionist in a bank, and kept active in church and community affairs. So far as I knew she was on no drugs that would harm the kidneys, and her symptoms didn't sound like a bladder infection.

Nor did Etta look that sick when she came hurrying into the hospital. Her husband was with her, but she had him wait in the lobby. When the patient and I were alone in the treatment room, she blurted out her problem. "Doctor, it's the color of my urine. You're going to think this is crazy, but it's turned blue!"

The nurse helped the patient get a sample of urine, and sure enough the urine was as blue as the autumn sky outside. I asked the patient if she had taken any medicines of any sort.

"Yes, my back started hurting day before yesterday, and I thought these would help." She produced a package of pills that were advertised for the relief of "nagging backache" and were obviously intended for people who thought that nagging backache meant a kidney problem. The pills, available without a prescription, did contain a mild pain reliever as well as a dye, methylene blue. This dye was what had changed the color of Etta's urine.

My patient grew angry with herself when I explained what had happened. "I should have called you in the first place!" she said. "But if it's not my kidneys, what's causing my back pain?"

I told the patient that we would go ahead and submit the urine sample for laboratory analysis to make sure that she didn't have an infection. Then I began questioning Etta about her activities, and she admitted having moved furniture the day before the backache began. My opinion was that she had experienced a mild back sprain. I went on to explain that the kidneys are very rarely the cause of back pain but that, anyway, the best way to treat the kidneys was not by taking drugs, but by using the least expensive medicine in the world.

"What is it?" Etta asked.

"Water," I told her.

Putting the Least Expensive Medicine to Work for You

Your kidneys are filters, and the more water and other fluids you drink, the better they can work to remove wastes from your bloodstream. Water is a tonic for the kidneys, and here are some guidelines on how much you need:

- *Drink at least a quart of water every day.*
- *The larger you are, the more water you need.*
- *The more active you are, the more water you need. During warm weather, you may need to drink two quarts or more a day.*
- *Learn to supplement your water intake by drinking juices, beverages, tea, and other liquids.*

- *If your urine remains yellow throughout the day, you aren't drinking enough water.*

The Natural Way Joe Discovered to Avoid Kidney Stones

Joe, a 48-year-old lineman, came to the hospital complaining of excruciating pain that would start in his back and penetrate all the way down to his groin. The pain was unbearable. Joe kept getting off the stretcher to hop around the room and cry out for relief. Finally a shot began to take hold, and the patient was admitted under the care of a surgeon. An x-ray showed that the problem was a kidney stone. It was lodged in one of the pencil-sized pipes that carries urine from the kidneys to the bladder. Joe suffered for two days before he passed the kidney stone, but at least he was spared from having an operation.

Before Joe left the hospital, the surgeon asked me to see if I could find the cause of the kidney stone. The patient was more than willing to help in the workup. "Anything," he told me. "I'll do anything to keep from having another kidney stone."

Certain of the body's processes can go wrong and cause a kidney stone to form, but all of Joe's tests checked out normal. This made me wonder if Joe wasn't getting enough water while at work. I asked him about it.

"Oh, I have coffee with breakfast," he said, "then nothing until lunch. At lunch I'll have another cup of coffee, and then at supper a glass of tea or two. That's about it."

"Nothing else?"

"Nope."

Joe described his urine as always being a dark yellow color, which meant to me that his kidneys were having to do the best they could on his very low intake of fluids. It was just the type of thing that favored a kidney stone. I pointed out that unless he changed his habits, Joe was likely to have another kidney stone, and another after that. He needed several times as much fluid as he had been getting, and this was the advice I gave him:

- Drink a large glass of juice and two cups of coffee at breakfast.
- Stop in midmorning and have a soft drink or glass of water.

- Have another soft drink with lunch. And drink one glass of water after finishing lunch.
- Stop in midafternoon for another soft drink or a large glass of water.
- Drink two large glasses of tea or water for supper.
- Drink a large glass of water an hour before bedtime.

Joe followed my advice and has not had another kidney stone in the three years since then.

Using Three Natural Antiseptics That Help to Cleanse the Urinary Tract

Germs that get into the bladder can cause a urine infection, but the body has some natural ways of defending against an infection. The most important one is the flushing action of urine as it passes out of the bladder. Three natural antiseptics that will help to cleanse the urine tract are:

1. *Water.* Drinking a lot of water will increase the volume of urine. This simple act alone will have an antiseptic effect, because as the urine flows from the bladder to the outside, it flushes out the germs that could cause an infection. The importance of this antiseptic action can be shown by the following case history.

Jane's Discovery of an Overlooked Way to Protect Her Bladder and Kidneys

Jane, a librarian, had always been bothered by bladder infections, and these became worse after she got married at the age of 46. "Honeymoon cystitis" was the name her doctor gave to the condition, but to Jane it was anything but a laughing matter to be bothered by burning on urination, frequent trips to the bathroom and the need to take two large white pills four times daily.

Women are more susceptible to bladder infections than men, and some women have more trouble than others. Jane was one of the susceptible ones, and the sexual activity she began to have after marriage had a tendency to introduce germs into the opening of her urine tract.

"One way you may be able to get by without having to take pills," her doctor told her, "is to make sure you go to the bathroom and pass urine after having sexual relations. And while you're in there, drink two big glasses of water or a soft drink. The extra fluid will force you to get up a time or two during the night, but if it keeps you from getting a bladder infection it may be worth it."

Jane followed the physician's advice. In the previous few months she had suffered through six bladder infections, but she had only one infection in the next year. She was careful to keep her water intake high all the time and to take the precautions the doctor had mentioned on those "special" nights.

2. *Cranberry juice.* Normal urine is slightly on the acid side, and this makes it harder for germs to grow. Cranberry juice adds to the acid content of urine, and drinking the juice can benefit the person who has frequent bladder infections. There is one problem. You need two or three large glasses of cranberry juice a day, and most people just don't want to drink that much of it. However, you can drink cranberry juice some of the time and use citrus fruits at other times.

3. *Citrus fruits.* Citrus fruits contain ascorbic acid, and this acid appears in the urine and acts as an antiseptic. The citrus fruits are oranges, grapefruit, lemons and limes. The usefulness of orange and grapefruit juice in holding down urinary infections was made apparent to me by a doctor who had a tendency to have kidney infections.

The Man Who Drank His Medicine Three Times a Day

Woody B. was a 60-year-old general practitioner with a tendency to develop kidney infections. In medical school 35 years previously he had his first kidney infection, and he had averaged about one infection a year until he began to take urinary antiseptics. Doctors can give pills that will increase the acid content of the urine, and for years and years Woody had been taking ascorbic acid in the form of vitamin-C tablets. He took eight tablets a day. Woody would have no doubt continued taking ascorbic acid but for the fact that he got an ulcer. I met him during his stay in the hospital.

"What I want you or one of the residents to tell me," he said, "is how I'm going to keep from getting kidney infections now that my ulcer diet strictly forbids me from taking those vitamin-C tablets."

I knew of several patients who drank cranberry juice to give the urine an antiseptic action and suggested this to the doctor. He frowned. "I don't like the taste of cranberry juice."

"Well, why don't you try eating citrus fruits—or drinking orange and grapefruit juice?"

"I'll give it a try," he said. "You get me started on it here in the hospital, and let's see how much good it does."

He began drinking three large glasses of orange or grapefruit juice a day, and the laboratory confirmed that his urine was staying well down in the acid range. Before he left the hospital, Woody shook my hand. "Drinking that juice is more fun than taking those pills anyway," he said. "And besides, one of the things I'm supposed to do is keep up a high fluid intake. Drinking that citrus juice kills two birds with one stone. I'm a believer in citrus juice now, and I don't think I'll have any more trouble with kidney infections."

A Good Practice for Anyone Who Desires Good Health

Taking foods and juices instead of pills is a good practice for anyone who desires good health. Physicians sometimes tend to forget that medicines began as extracts from plants or as potions made from natural ingredients. Natural remedies are still the best! What could be more natural than water, or using foods such as cranberry juice or the citrus fruits?

One problem that unfortunately seems to be increasing is that of drug-induced kidney damage. Many of the drugs that physicians prescribe have the potential of damaging the kidneys. A partial list of these drugs includes:

- Streptomycin
- Kanamycin
- Neomycin
- Colymycin
- Polymyxin B
- Vancomycin
- Gentamicin
- Amphotericin B
- Gold salts
- Phenacetin

Your best protection against receiving these and other drugs that can damage your kidneys is to choose a physician who is willing to discuss the good *and* bad effects of every drug and to search with you for a drug that is least likely to cause serious side effects. Still, the best medicine for the kidneys is the least expensive, and it is also the safest. And by using water in the right doses, you just may be able to avoid having any kidney problems at all.

The Diet That Can Take a Load off the Kidneys

Some persons do develop a degree of kidney failure, and diet is one of the best treatments for this condition. In the first place, if you have been told by your physician that you have mild kidney failure, you can't drink all the fluid you want. How much you *can* drink will depend on the function of your kidneys and on what your doctor tells you. The general guide is to drink less water if you note a rapid weight gain or develop swelling of the legs or feet. You should also avoid eating a lot of meat and go easy on dairy products, which are high in phosphorus. The following diet is one that can serve as a guideline for the person with mild kidney failure. The diet takes a load off your kidneys by keeping to a minimum the things that a diseased kidney is least able to excrete:

BREAKFAST

    ½ cup orange juice
    1 soft-cooked egg
    1 cup cereal
    coffee or tea with sugar

LUNCH

    1 slice whole wheat bread
    1 cup shredded lettuce
    oil & vinegar
    ½ cup applesauce
    1 ounce American cheese

SUPPER

    1 ounce of lean meat

½ cup canned green beans
½ cup mashed potatoes
2 peach halves
2 teaspoons of unsaturated margarine
coffee or tea with sugar

SNACKS

Hard candies, marshmellows, jelly beans and gumdrops

Eating Right to Avoid the Symptoms of Disease

To someone with mild kidney failure, a diet like the one above can mean the difference between feeling well and being sick. Colleen C., a 50-year-old woman, was extremely ill on admission to the hospital. She had been vomiting for two days, and collapsed in her home; an ambulance rushed her to the emergency room. We could barely rouse her, and she answered questions incoherently. Lab tests quickly confirmed my clinical diagnosis of kidney failure. The patient's BUN level was 190 mg%. The BUN is a test of kidney function, and the normal level of this blood chemical should not exceed 20 mg%.

I gave the patient intravenous fluid therapy, and when she was well enough to eat I put her on a diet that was low in meats and dairy products and high in fruits and vegetables and fats. She thrived on the diet, and her BUN fell to near normal. Further studies showed that for many years, Colleen had a low-grade kidney infection; she was prone to attacks of kidney failure when the infection worsened or when she ate a lot of meat and dairy products.

Said she: "I didn't know for sure that what I was eating could make me sick, but I can remember feeling nauseated after a steak. Another thing was that I always got sicker than everybody else. One little virus would wipe me out, especially if I got sick at the stomach and couldn't drink any water."

Colleen took medicine to prevent another kidney infection, and she also went on a diet. During the time I followed her, she had no more trouble with kidney failure. She did get nauseous for several days when she stopped taking in any salt. She read in a magazine about the benefits of a low-salt diet, which were discussed in Chapter 4 of this book. They didn't say in the article something I am going to say now. Listen carefully, because this advice could be important. *If you have mild kidney failure, do not go on a low-salt diet unless your doctor tells you to do so.* Your body needs more salt than a low-salt diet can give, and restricting salt can make you sick. The important thing if you have kidney disease is to follow your doctor's directions closely. And be sure to go in for regular medical check-ups.

9

Natural Ways to Keep Your Digestive Tract Healthy and Comfortable

We Americans spend over a million dollars a year on laxatives, and even more than this on medicines for heartburn, indigestion, diarrhea, and other intestinal symptoms. Most of these medicines are unnecessary. By following a few simple rules, you can keep your digestive tract at its peak of health and feel younger by enjoying normal digestive processes.

Here are five ways to have normal bowel movements *without the need for laxatives:*

1. *Stop taking laxatives.*
2. *Drink plenty of fluids.*
3. *Develop a regular bowel habit.*
4. *Eat food laxatives.*
5. *Exercise every day.*

How Jean A. Kicked the Laxative Habit by Using the Best Medicine of All

Jean, a 55-year-old housewife, was a little upset that I didn't want to renew her prescription for a laxative. I was pinch-hitting for her regular physician, and he had been prescribing this same medicine for years.

"Why can't I have it?" the patient asked.

"You don't need it," I told her. "I've just examined you and you're in good health, and that means you can have normal bowel movements without using laxatives."

The patient gave me a cool look. "But I need something to help," she said.

"I didn't say you didn't need help, just that you didn't need to take laxatives." I explained to Jean that the body has a natural mechanism for causing a bowel movement every day or so. "When you fill your stomach with food, reflexes go to your lower intestine to cause squeezing actions. You feel these and know it's time for a bowel movement. But when you use a laxative, it goes against your natural reflexes."

The patient thought about it and asked, "You mean that using a laxative makes me dependent on it?"

I said yes. In the ensuing discussion I realized that Jean took laxatives not only because they were a habit, but because she failed to do many of the things that were necessary to have normal bowel action. She didn't drink enough water, she didn't exercise, and she didn't eat food laxatives. Also, Jean was worried that she might go an entire day without having a bowel movement. I explained that she could go one, two or three days without a bowel movement, even a week, and nothing bad would happen to her. Here is the program I recommended for her:

FIRST WEEK

1. Cut the dose of laxative in half.
2. Drink six glasses of water a day.
3. Heed any call to stool by going to the bathroom and trying to have a bowel movement.

SECOND WEEK

1. Stop the laxative.
2. Continue the high fluid intake.
3. Exercise three times a day.
4. Concentrate on eating food laxatives.
5. Continue efforts to have regular bowel movements.

I didn't see Jean again, but I did talk to her physician a few months later. I asked how the patient was doing and was pleased to hear that she had stopped the laxatives and was getting by the natural way. The doctor laughed and said, "I know that water is the best medicine to keep the bowels working normally, but I have to admit that when people ask me for a laxative it's easier just to give it to them than to explain why they don't need it. But I'm glad you took the trouble to help Jean."

Drinking Your Way to the Healthy, Natural Rhythm

About four-fifths of the water you drink is absorbed before it reaches the lower part of the colon. But if you let your fluid intake get too low, even less of the water you drink reaches the rectum. Water is a natural lubricant, and without it the stool can become hard and difficult to pass. Drink at least six eight-ounce glasses of fluid a day, and drink more than this if the weather is hot and you perspire heavily. Some people find that warm water first thing in the morning is a natural laxative. "I drink a big cup of warm water first thing in the morning," one man told me, "and it's the quickest-acting laxative in the world!" Others find that coffee or hot tea acts the same way.

The Advantages of Doing Things the Regular Way

Breaking a laxative habit isn't easy, but it can be done. Don't stop taking your laxative suddenly. Spend two weeks cutting down on the dosage and then cutting it out completely. Increase your water intake during this time and begin to cultivate a normal bowel habit. You don't have to have a bowel movement every day. Perhaps every other day is natural for you. At any rate, select a time after one of your meals and visit the bathroom. Most people develop the habit for right after breakfast, to take advantage of the digestive processes that occurred during the night, but you can be just as happy and healthy with a bowel movement after supper or following the noon meal. Just heed your body and listen to its urges. When you feel the least stirrings that point to the need for a bowel movement, visit the bathroom!

Once there, relax. Don't force things. Plan to spend at least 15 minutes performing this important body function. Squatting is the best position to pass stool, but commodes don't take this into account. You may find that it helps for you to plant your feet on a stool in front of the commode or to bend forward so that your abdomen rests against your thighs.

Remember, if you need some help while you are recovering your natural habit, give yourself a tap water enema. The enema helps to remove stool from the lowest part of the colon. A laxative, by contrast, upsets the rhythm of the entire intestinal tract.

Enjoying the Benefits of Food Laxatives

You can choose from many foods that have a laxative effect. Some foods stimulate muscular actions in the intestinal tract, while other foods promote normal movements by increasing the roughage content of the bowel.

- FOODS THAT STIMULATE INTESTINAL ACTION:

Prunes	Blackberries	Wheat germ
Bananas	Figs	Rice
Apples	Pears	Grains
Apricots	Peaches	Pumpkin

- FOODS THAT PROMOTE NORMALITY BY RAISING THE ROUGHAGE CONTENT OF THE BOWEL:

Lettuce	Mustard greens	String beans
Cabbage	Brussels sprouts	Bean sprouts
Spinach	Broccoli	Asparagus
Sweet potatoes	Tomatoes	Peas

These foods promote normal bowel movements, and they are nutritious, too. Eating them keeps your digestive processes working smoothly and at the same time provides your body the raw, wholesome ingredients it needs for good health!

How Royce Discovered That One Thing Can Make All the Difference in Having Normal Bowel Movements or Being Constipated

Royce M., a 44-year-old construction worker, needed surgery when he broke his hip in an accident. He was forced to lie in bed in traction after the operation, and he got something he hadn't expected: constipation.

"I've never had this," he told me. "I guess it was because of working from morning till night, but I was regular as clockwork. Now I have to take an enema to do what used to come naturally."

I told him not to fret, that his problem was temporary. "It's lying in bed all day without any exercise. But you'll get your regularity back as soon as you get on your feet again."

Taking Full Advantage of Body Movement

Like Royce, many people are constipated because of a lack of activity. If you are confined to a bed or a wheelchair that is one thing, but if you are able to move around and yet don't, that is something else. The simple fact is this: The more you use your body, the less trouble you will have with constipation. Here are two rules to follow:

Rule 1. Do exercises that strengthen your abdominal muscles. Lie on your back on a hard surface. Raise both legs slowly until they are perpendicular to the ground. Return them to the resting position. Repeat the exercise several times. This exercise is explained more fully in Chapter 4. It strengthens your abdominal muscles and makes it easier to have normal bowel movements.

Rule 2. Walk at least 15 or 20 minutes every day. Walking every day is the one thing that can make all the difference in having normal bowel movements or being constipated. Do other activities help? Certainly! Working in the yard, running errands, doing housework, doing manual labor—all these count. But for most people walking is the best way to ensure having normal bowel movements. And walking can have additional benefits.

How Ruth C. Got Relief from Gas and Heartburn by Using a Safe and Simple Remedy

Ruth C. was bothered by belching and by an uncomfortable, burning sensation that came on about 20 minutes after she ate. She tried lying down after meals, but that made the problem worse. She tried taking an antacid, but it didn't give her complete relief. She came to the clinic because she was convinced she had an ulcer.

The studies and medical examination showed that Ruth had simple heartburn, or *peptic esophagitis.* Stomach acid would get into her gullet after she ate, and the irritation caused bloating and burning discomfort. I told Ruth that lying down right after a meal was the worst thing she could do, since that merely made it easier for the acid to leak back into her food passageway. Sitting down right after a meal was also bad, because it made her tummy push against her chest. What she needed to do, I explained, was to take a 20-minute walk after each meal. This would give her food a chance to settle and keep the stomach juices out of her gullet. Ruth took my advice and has had very little trouble with gas or heartburn since then.

Four Ways to Overcome Peptic Esophagitis

If you have belching, burning pain or a sourness in your stomach right after eating, you may have peptic esophagitis. You can do four things to overcome these symptoms:

#1. *Take a walk after your meals.* This is the way Ruth C. and so many others have overcome heartburn and indigestion. The walk will let your food settle and help to keep acid out of your food passageway.

#2. *Eat small meals.* You probably have most of your trouble after eating a big meal. The more food you eat, the more your stomach must expand. The bigger your stomach gets, the easier it is for stomach acid to boil up into your gullet and cause heartburn. What this means is that you need to keep your meals small. Spread your eating out into three or four small meals, and your symptoms will either disappear or lessen.

#3. *Lose weight.* An overweight person with heartburn can expect to have less trouble after reducing to his ideal weight (see Chapter 6).

#4. *Use antacids if the symptoms persist.* By neutralizing stomach juices, antacids can help to relieve heartburn. If

your heartburn is very troublesome you should be checked by your doctor; the physician can recommend a specific antacid. On the other hand, antacids are available without a prescription, and if you are going to take them you should know something about them.

Choosing the Antacid Therapy That Is Right for You

An antacid is a drug that reduces stomach acidity. It does not completely neutralize the stomach juices, because stomach acid is very potent, and its action is needed for normal digestion. What the antacid does is to take the edge off the acid and keep to a minimum the damage it can do if it gets into your esophagus. Some antacids are better than others, but the ones you hear the most about are not necessarily the best. Doctors tend to recommend one of the following antacids, and you can buy these in the drugstore without a prescription:

- *Gelusil®*. It comes in liquid or tablets, and the dosage is given on the label. Most patients prefer to take Gelusil® because they like the taste. It has the unfortunate side effect of making you constipated.
- *Maalox®*. Maalox® also comes in liquid or tablets, and because it contains magnesium hydroxide it has a tendency to make the bowels loose. To have normal bowel movements, use Gelusil® part of the time and Maalox® part of the time.
- *Trisogel®*. This antacid contains a mixture of ingredients that can prevent constipation or loose stools. It comes in liquid or tablets and has a fresh mint flavor.
- *Riopan®*. This antacid comes in tablets or liquid and has the advantage of being low in salt content. It is recommended for persons who have high blood pressure, heart disease, swelling of the feet or any condition that calls for a low-salt diet.

Remember that an antacid works best when you take it about one hour after eating. Until then, the food that you ate tended to neutralize the stomach acid. Finally, don't use the antacid if you have no symptoms and don't feel a need for it.

The Best Way to Control an Ulcer

A stomach or duodenal ulcer can be serious. It can bleed, eat through the lining of the stomach, or form a roadblock to keep food from getting into the intestine. A doctor can make the diagnosis and prescribe treatment, but in the last few years some interesting things about ulcer have come to light. I spent months of my specialty training learning about ulcer diets, ulcer drugs, and the indications for surgery on an ulcer patient. Now it appears that I was missing the point. Studies have shown that the main benefit of hospital treatment is the hospital itself! Putting someone to bed gets him out of the nerve-racking pace that caused the ulcer, and this alone is enough to produce healing.

The Thing John B. Did to Cure His Ulcer

John B., a salesman who was happy in his job, needed some extra money. Two of his children were about to enter college, prices had gone way up, and the family budget was stretched. For some time, John's boss had been urging him to take the job of regional sales manager. John had refused, because becoming an executive would make him responsible for ten other salesmen besides himself. Still, the promotion meant an increase in salary, and John finally decided to take the job.

For several weeks things went well. John worked much harder, but enjoyed the challenge. Then, the hardships of executive life began to occur. A man was found cheating on his sales and had to be fired. The firm began to lose some of their customers due to the introduction of a less expensive, foreign-made appliance. Gas and oil prices surged upward, and John had to justify why his salesmen spent so much money traveling, yet still weren't breaking any sales records.

One morning John woke up feeling nauseous. He stumbled into the bathroom and threw up. The vomitus had a coffee-grounds appearance, and on hearing this John's doctor told him to get in an ambulance and come straight to the hospital. Tests confirmed that John had a bleeding ulcer. Fortunately he did not bleed enough to require transfusions, but his blood count did drop and he had to be watched closely for several days.

The thing that was interesting about John, though, was how

much better he felt after just two days in the hospital. No, he didn't exactly remember a pain in his stomach, but there had been a tightness, a knot. "The funny thing is that I had to come into the hospital to realize that that knot's been with me ever since I took that regional sales manager job. My stomach feels better than it has in three and a half months."

The doctor explained that the important thing about an ulcer is "not what's eating your stomach, but what's eating you." In John's case, the answer was obvious: the new job. The patient had a choice: Change jobs or continue to have an ulcer. John made the right choice. He gave up the executive position, returned to the lower-paying but healthier job of salesman, and has had no more trouble with an ulcer.

Three Ways to Have a Healthier Stomach

You can take advantage of what John B. learned, and you can do so without waiting until you develop an ulcer. The three ways to have a healthier stomach are:

One.   *Don't drive yourself to do more than you can do.* If you're under too much pressure, you know it. Do something about it *before* you get sick. The mind affects the body! Nervous tension causes your stomach to make more acid, and the acid can give you an ulcer. No matter what your job or goal, your chances of success are much greater if you keep your health!

Two.   *Eat regular, nutritious meals.* Many doctors no longer believe that milk and milk products are the best diet for an ulcer patient. Instead, they recommend three nutritious meals a day. Try to eat your meals at about the same time each day, and don't skip meals. Your stomach will get used to receiving food at regular hours, and to miss a meal is to invite stomach acid to stir around and brew up trouble for you.

Three.   *Avoid eating things that can harm the stomach.* To have a stomach you can put just about anything in, don't put just anything into your stomach. Things to stay away from include alcohol and coffee in more than moderate quantities. Take coffee or alcohol with the meal or afterwards, so that the food will help to protect the stomach from any injurious effects. Aspirin and vitamin-C tablets can also harm the stomach. If you take either of these medicines, do so on a full stomach. Finally, smoking increases stomach acidity. Which is just one more reason for quitting this habit.

The Painless Way of Warding Off Attacks of "Colitis"

The person who suffers from an "irritable colon" or "spastic colitis" can take comfort from knowing that his bowel is not actually diseased. It is just very sensitive and may act up when the person eats certain foods. On the other hand, not eating the foods that cause diarrhea is a way of warding off the attacks of irritable colon. It comes down to making a choice between eating something you love and having diarrhea or not eating it and staying well.

How Wesley Learned to Avoid His Attacks of Diarrhea

Wesley, a 60-year-old retired fireman, had been bothered by attacks of pain and diarrhea. He sought medical help, and I made a diagnosis of irritable colon. "Now," I told the patient, "let's make a list of foods that cause the attacks, and then you can prevent the diarrhea by staying away from them."

"Corn is the main thing, doctor, and then there's anything with celery. Beans do it. Mexican food . . . ." He went on to name the foods that were giving him trouble. I suggested he remove these items from his diet.

However, Wesley continued to have attacks of diarrhea and belly pain. We eliminated more foods. The attacks continued. Perhaps they would be occurring yet, but for something the patient's wife told me. It was during a particularly bad attack, after I saw Wesley in the emergency room. The nurse gave him something for pain, and I stepped into the hall to speak to his wife. "What did he eat for supper?" I asked her.

"Corn," she said without batting an eye.

"But he's not supposed to eat corn! It's not on his diet."

"Doctor, he's been eating it right along. Never did give it up."

When I confronted the patient with this, he did not deny it. "I know you said to cut it out, and I did cut those other things out. But corn: It's my favorite food. Until tonight, I thought I'd rather have diarrhea than give up corn. But this attack has made a believer out of me."

Wesley's failure to follow his diet caused more than just an attack of diarrhea and belly pain. His loose bowels caused his hemorrhoids to start bleeding, and he had to have surgery. He was in the hospital for three weeks, but I can assure you that he did eliminate corn from his diet when he returned home.

The food that bothers you may not be corn. It may be a certain spice, or mushrooms, or lasagna, or a favorite dessert. Once you determine what causes your abdominal pain or diarrhea, the treatment is simple: Eliminate that food from your diet.

Natural Ways to Treat Diarrhea

Diarrhea is usually self-limiting. Medicine you're taking may cause it, or the diarrhea may accompany the intestinal flu. Bed rest is indicated if you have severe diarrhea. Usually by the next day you'll be able to get around and take liquids. To give your system time to recover, eat soft foods before going back to regular table fare. Or, choose foods that help to relieve diarrhea. Among these are:

Ice cream	Peanut butter and toast
Cheese	Eggs, soft boiled
Rice pudding	Bread pudding
Creamed chicken	Custard

Remember that if an attack of diarrhea persists, call your physician. He will try to find out what's wrong and treat the underlying cause. Should you have fever with your diarrhea or see blood or mucous in your stool, call the physician immediately.

10

Keeping Your Skin
Young and Alive
by Using Natural Remedies

Your skin is the most visible part of you. It is a mirror that reflects your health, and it tends to sprout wrinkles and become dry as you grow older. You can't stop the relentless advance of time, but you can do some things that will keep your skin at its youngest, healthiest efficiency. You can also take advantage of an overlooked way to slow the development of wrinkles and skin creases. Here are some ways to keep your skin young and alive:

#1. Let your skin take care of itself. Don't doctor it with chemicals such as strong deodorants, antiperspirants or "antibacterial" soap. It's normal for bacteria to live on your skin, and there's no need to get rid of them.

#2. Bathe regularly using mild soap. The natural way to control skin odor is to bathe! If odor indicates the need, bathe once daily—more often if you have been working heavily and want to feel clean and fresh. On the other hand, many people are happy to get by with a bath every second or third day. Use the mildest, simplest soap you can find.

#3. Use your fingers to clean your skin. You don't need to bathe with a bath rag or sponge, and this is especially true if your skin is dry or sensitive. Use your fingers to apply the soap and lather, and go easy. Light cleansing is as

good as hard scrubbing and isn't nearly so damaging to the skin.

#4. Practice drying the soothing way. If your skin is dry or sensitive, learn to blot yourself dry instead of rubbing your skin vigorously with a towel. A gentle blotting motion is easier on the skin. Even more soothing is to stand and drip dry or let a fan blow on your wet skin and speed the drying process.

#5. Protect your skin from things that can harm it. You may have an allergy to clothing or to something in your diet. Learn to avoid what hurts your skin, and remember that the sun is more harmful than just about anything else except fire. And actually, the sun *is* fire: It burns the skin. Perhaps the worst thing about getting too much sun is that it makes you look old.

Fay's Discovery of a Way to Keep Her Skin Young

Fay, a 45-year-old socialite, woke up one morning, looked at herself in the mirror—and saw wrinkles! She had lived an active life, working in community projects, playing lots of tennis, enjoying a swim every day in the warm months. Each summer she and her husband flew to Europe, and each winter they took at least one skiing vacation to Colorado. The only thing Fay had not done in her first 45 years was take care of her skin. She had a lovely tan, but the wrinkles were there, no doubt about that.

"I can't promise those wrinkles will go away," her physician told her, "but I can tell you the best way to keep any more of them from coming. And that is simply to stay out of the sun. And if you do go outdoors, wear a hat, cover yourself with clothing, and use a sunscreen on your forehead, cheeks and hands."

The physician went on to explain that all those suntans Fay had enjoyed through the years had prematurely aged her skin. And why not? Sun damages the skin, and a much-admired suntan is really just a scar that forms in response to sun injury. The physician who presented Fay's case at a medical meeting did not go so far as to say that the crow's-feet around the patient's eyes had disappeared since she began avoiding the sun, but he did say that his patient's face looked fresher and younger after she began protecting herself from the sun.

Putting Fay's Method to Work for You

The three things Fay's doctor recommended for her were designed to protect her skin from the sun. You can use these same methods to keep your own skin young and wrinkle free:

1. *Avoid the sun when possible.* A little sun won't hurt you, but going out of your way to get a suntan is neither healthy nor wise. Your ordinary exercising will give you enough sun for your skin to manufacture vitamin D. Beyond that, excessive exposure to the sun damages your skin. Unfortunately, the damage builds up as you grow older; the more sun you get, the greater are your chances later in life of developing skin cancer.

2. *Wear protective clothing.* Wear a hat to protect your face from the sun. Select light-colored clothing that completely protects the back and arms and neck and legs. It's okay to wear short sleeves when the weather is hot, but be sure that you

3. *Use a sunscreen over exposed parts of your skin.* Use a sunscreen when your skin is exposed to the sun for more than 15 or 20 minutes at a time; as a general rule, the lighter your skin color the more you need the protection offered by a sunscreen. Almost any oily substance will provide some protection from the sun. You can use plain petrolatum or red petrolatum, or choose a skin cream that contains zinc oxide or kaolin. Many commercial sunscreens are available, and probably the most effective ones are those that contain para-aminobenzoic acid. PreSun® is one such product. If you are prone to have skin allergies, use cold cream as your sunscreen.

How Vicki Relieved the Itching and Flaking of Dry Skin

Vicki S., a 50-year-old physical therapist, was bothered by dry, flaky skin. What was especially aggravating, she told me, was the itching. "It seems like once I get started scratching my hands or arms, they just go on and on itching, and pretty soon the skin is so raw it looks like it'll bleed if I touch it. And yet it still itches!"

Dry skin tends to itch, and scratching can make the skin angry and create a maddening desire to keep on scratching. Doctors call this the "itch-scratch cycle," because the more you scratch, the more you itch. The best way to get relief is to find out what caused the itching in the first place and do something about it. In Vicki's case, the problem was wetness. Nothing can dry out the skin more quickly than water. As a physical therapist, Vicki had to put her hands and arms in and out of whirlpool baths, and she also found it necessary to wash her hands frequently. All this wetness led to dry skin—and furious itching. The things that worked to relieve Vicki's problem can also work for you:

Three Ways to Relieve the Symptoms of Dry Skin

1. *Avoid bathing too often or for too long.* Regular bathing is a desirable habit, but if you have dry skin you should limit yourself to one bath a day and keep it to less than half an hour. Because water and soap wash away natural skin oils, bathing can add to the dryness of skin. This is especially true during the winter months.

2. *Wear comfortable clothing.* Dry skin is sensitive! Keep irritation to a minimum by wearing loose-fitting, comfortable cotton garments. Cotton is soft, and it is easier on your skin than nylon, wool or other fabrics. Choose clothing that doesn't need starch, and wash the garment frequently. The older it gets the better it will feel on your skin.

3. *Add a soothing oil to your skin once a day.* The best time to apply skin oil is right after a bath. Using your fingers, apply a light coating of Alpha-Keri®, Nivea® skin oil, Lubath® or a similar product to your skin. Olive oil is an inexpensive and excellent treatment for dry skin. Buy it right off the grocer's shelf. One product may appeal to you more than another, and in fact, one skin oil may work better for you than it does for someone else. Some agents, such as Alpha-Keri®, can be added to the bath. However, the oil causes rings around the tub, and unless these are washed away the bath will be oily for the next person, who may not wish it to be.

How Lareina Learned That Natural
Skin Care Is the Best Skin Care

Lareina R., a housewife and mother of two teen-aged sons, came to the emergency room for a distressing and embarrassing problem. The skin of her armpits was red and swollen, and itched so intensely that in several spots she had scratched it until it bled. She could barely stand to keep her arms down in their regular position.

The location of the rash was unusual. However, its location can suggest the cause of a skin problem. Bumps that affect only the ankles and lower legs, for example, suggest insect bites; a rash on the hands suggests an allergy to gloves or to something the person touched. Hearing that Lareina had two teen-aged sons, I made a guess as to what had happened, and my guess turned out to be correct. I asked the patient if she had sprayed her underarms with anything unusual in the last few days.

"Yes, come to think of it I have. Bill, my oldest, kept talking about how good this new antiperspirant was, so I tried it out the night before last."

"And when did the rash begin?"

"Yesterday."

What Lareina had was an allergic reaction to the antiperspirant. Tactfully, I tried to point out that in my opinion she didn't really need to use such products. "They don't really keep you from sweating, and there's no need to keep from sweating anyway. Sweating is natural. Bathing and changing clothes is the solution."

Needless to say, the patient was more than happy to follow my suggestion and stay away from underarm sprays. She also had to give herself a week of close skin care to get over the rash.

How to Avoid the Things That Harm Your Skin

Lareina's reaction to the antiperspirant convinced her that she shouldn't spray her skin with similar products. She found out the hard way that just because a product is made doesn't mean that it is safe to use. A few years ago, for example, feminine hygiene sprays were put on the market. These products are unnecessary in the first place and can actually cause harm to the user by creating an allergic reaction. Probably the most common things that cause skin allergies are soaps, detergents and cleaning agents used in the kitchen or bathroom. Cosmetics run these a close second. You can use hypoallergenic cosmetics, ones that are least likely to cause an allergic reaction, and if your hands are sensitive you should wear protective rubber or plastic gloves when using soaps or detergents. The best way to prevent an allergy, in other words, is to avoid coming in contact with the substance that causes it. Sometimes the allergen is something outside the house, either in the yard or the woods, and to avoid it takes special care.

The Trick Homer R. Used
to Keep from Getting Poison Ivy

Homer developed severe itching on his hands and ankles after working in the yard. The red scratches and weeping from the rash told me instantly that it was poison ivy. "I don't care what it is," Homer said. "Just give me something to cure it."

I told the patient that I could prescribe some medicine to help out on the itching, but that I couldn't "cure" the rash. It would take about two weeks for the symptoms to go away, even with treatment. "Mr. R.," I told the patient, "the only cure for a poison ivy allergy is to keep from coming in contact with the plant. And to do that, you have to learn what it looks like and stay away from it."

It turned out that Homer and his wife had recently moved into a new house, and it was located in the suburbs among the trees, shrubbery and poison ivy. The patient checked a book on plants out of the library, learned to recognize poison ivy, and has had no further trouble with this allergy.

How to Save Yourself Two Weeks of Itching

You, too, can profit from knowing how to recognize poison ivy, poison oak and poison sumac. These plants are not really "poison." They do contain an oil that can cause your skin to break out after you touch the plant. Some people are more sensitive than others, and these persons must be especially careful when walking through the woods. Here are some ways to save yourself two weeks of itching:

1. *Learn to recognize poison ivy, poison oak and poison sumac, and stay away from them.* Not all of these plants may grow where you live. If you reside in Texas, for instance, poison ivy and poison sumac are the two plants you have to avoid. Poison oak is much more of a problem in California. Florida and other states in the deep south are apt to have all three plants.

2. *Remember that you can contact the plant without directly touching it.* The oil from poison ivy can get on shoes, auto tires and clothing, and may reach your skin when you handle these items. Wear old clothes when you go into dense woods; wash them out as soon as you're back home. Another way you can get the rash is to pet an animal that has come in contact with the plant. It may be a good idea to keep the pet at home until you can find out where it brushed against the poison ivy. You may be surprised to find that the plant is growing in your back yard!

3. *You may prevent the allergy by washing your hands after touching the plant.* However, for washing to work you have to remove the oil within five or ten minutes after it gets on your skin.

4. *You may be able to protect your skin when exposure to the plant is inevitable.* Wear gloves and long sleeves. Put a paste of soap and water on your wrists or any other exposed part of your body. The soap will shield you and make it easier to wash the oils off.

What to Do When Itching Does Occur

The treatment for any skin allergy is to remove the cause and clear up the symptoms. Here are some ways to get relief:

1. *The wetter the rash, the wetter the remedy.* Whether or not you scratch it, skin rash can ooze fluid. The natural tendency is to put powder or some other dry substance on the wet skin. Don't! Use soaks to treat a wet rash, because they will dry it more quickly than any other form of treatment. Here are some soaks you can use:

- *Salt and water.* Add two teaspoons of salt to a quart of water.
- *Soda and water.* Add eight teaspoons of baking soda to a quart of water.
- *Burow's soaks.* Buy some Domeboro® powder or tablets at the drugstore. Drop one or two packets or tablets into a pint of water and stir.

Apply the liquid to the rash with a soft cotton rag. Torn pieces of a sheet or pillowcase are ideal. Begin by dipping the rag in the soak and then keep the rag moist by pouring small amounts of the soak on it. Use the soaks three or four times a day until the rash dries up. You'll find that intense itching goes away following the use of a soak.

2. *Use calamine lotion for the relief of itching.* This product is safe and effective and can be bought without a prescription. Use plain calamine lotion, because the product containing Benadryl® can cause an allergic skin rash. Be sure to gently wash the old calamine off before applying a new coat of medicine. It's best not to use calamine lotion on a wet, weeping rash. Use soaks until your skin has dried and then apply the calamine.

3. *Baby your skin until the rash wears off.* Don't rub the inflamed skin vigorously with a towel. Blot it dry or let it air dry. Wear soft cotton garments over the rash and sleep on soft cotton bed linens. Try to avoid scratching the rash, and cut your nails if you have an irresistible urge to scratch. After the rash has begun to heal, a light coating of Alpha-Keri® or other skin oil may reduce the amount of itching.

Choosing Your Skin Care as You Eat

Food allergies can cause blotches of red, itchy hives to break out on the body, and the reaction may cause nausea and fever. Foods that can provoke a reaction in a susceptible person include wheat, eggs, milk, strawberries and chocolate. The best treatment is to identify the offending food and eliminate it from the diet (see Chapter 3). Hives usually don't last long, but if they are uncomfortable you should see a doctor.

Sometimes the problem is not a food allergy, but a reaction to a medicine the person has taken.

The Man Who Took Something for Headache and Ended Up in the Hospital

Merle S. was gasping for air. His blood pressure was dangerously low, his body was covered with red whelps, and he was wheezing. I knew that he either had asthma or an allergic reaction, and the emergency treatment was the same. I injected adrenaline deep into the muscles of his arm and gave him a good dose of steroid hormones in the veins. Within 5 minutes after he'd arrived in the emergency room, Merle was breathing easier.

"Do you have asthma?" I asked.

"No, but I'm allergic to aspirin."

"Did you take some?"

He nodded and began shivering. His wife had been standing by, and she stepped forward. "He had a headache, and took that _____you see advertised on television. We didn't know it had aspirin in it. About 15 minutes later he started breaking out with hives, and I called the ambulance when he began having trouble breathing."

Prompt treatment saved Merle's life, but he could have avoided the reaction if he'd been more careful about the medicine he took. Merle was in the hospital a week, and his doctor told me they had worked out a new system for avoiding allergic reactions. Merle was not to take *anything* without first checking with the doctor. Not bad advice for a person with allergies.

Keeping Away from Drugs That Can Harm You

If you have a drug allergy, you know to stay away from that drug. Be sure, as well, to avoid using similar products that may contain the unwanted compound. Here are the medicines that cause most of the allergic drug reactions:

- Penicillin
- Aspirin
- Narcotics (pain killers)
- Iodides
- Tetracycline and other antibiotics

Make sure your physician knows about your allergies, and if the allergy is severe, you may want to wear a bracelet stating this fact. This way, if you are unable to speak for yourself (after a severe injury, for example) the people taking care of you will know of the allergy. You can order a bracelet from the Medic Alert Foundation, P.O. Box 1009, Turlock, California 95380. Medic Alert is a non-profit organization that was founded after a doctor's daughter almost died from a reaction to a serum injection (she was allergic to the serum yet was unable after her injury to tell the attending physician about the allergy). In addition to listing your allergy, the bracelet will have the phone number of a Central Registry. By calling this number, a physician can get the details of your past medical history.

11

Natural Ways That Will
Free You from Headache

Headache is that most human of miseries. Many things can cause it, and most of us have experienced the discomfort of a headache at one time or other. When headaches become a problem, it's time to do something about them. Chances are very good that you can free yourself from headache by following the advice in this chapter. The three general guidelines that will help you to overcome headache are:

1. Find the cause of the headache.
2. Eliminate that cause to prevent the headache.
3. Use natural treatments to stop headaches when they occur.

How Sylvia Got Relief by Getting to the Bottom of Her Problem

Sylvia had always taken aspirin for her headaches, but the aspirin began to cause severe indigestion, and she thought she might be getting an ulcer. She did not have an ulcer, but she was right in wanting to avoid the very harmful side effects that can occur when one takes aspirin all the time.

"Did you ever try to find the cause of your headaches?" I asked her as she was leaving the office.

She smiled. "No, but I've been told they were probably tension headaches. The only thing wrong with that is I'm not a very tense person."

I had a suggestion for her. "Sylvia, I want you to start keeping a record of your headaches. Bring the record back in two weeks, and let's see if we can learn anything."

I went on to explain that keeping a record of the headaches would help in getting to the bottom of what was causing them. Here are some of the things I suggested the patient do:

- *Note the time of day when a headache occurs.*
- *Note how long the headache lasts.*
- *Record other symptoms such as nausea or dizziness.*
- *Write down everything that happened in the hour preceding the headache.*

Sylvia's "headache record" was very interesting. She had headaches twice a day, around noon and an hour or two after supper. The thing that was common to both times was that she was watching television. One other thing that seemed to bring on the headaches was reading a magazine. "You know, it's funny," she said, "but they do occur when I'm using my eyes, especially if I'm already kind of tired." Sylvia's headache record suggested that she was suffering from eyestrain. She visited an eye doctor, obtained glasses, and stopped having headaches!

Finding the Cause Is the First Step to Curing the Headache

It isn't always easy to find the cause of headaches. However, most ordinary headaches are caused by only a few conditions. By keeping a headache record, you can tell if your problem is due to one of the common conditions. Here are the most frequent types of headache and the symptoms of each condition:

1. *Tension headache.* This is the most common type of headache, and painful spasm of the muscles at the back of the neck causes it. Sometimes tender lumps or bumps appear in these muscles. The headaches are brought on by tension, worry, anger or frustration.

2. *Eyestrain.* Pain in the forehead is the body's way of telling you that you've strained your eyes while reading, sewing, watching television or doing close work such as bookkeep-

ing. The headache will go away when you rest your eyes for an hour or two.

3. *Lack of sleep.* This headache follows a restless night or a night's sleep that wasn't long enough. The symptoms may be the same as eyestrain, or pain can occur in any part of the head. A nap or normal night's rest will relieve the headache.

4. *Hangover headache.* The "morning after" headache gets most of its publicity for occurring after a night of heavy drinking. However, it can follow the use of tranquilizers, sleeping pills or other drugs. It is usually present on awakening or soon after and tends to go away by noon.

5. *Food allergy.* You get the headache of food allergy by eating the causative food. The headache may be accompanied by other symptoms, including nausea, dizziness, skin rash and drainage of mucous from the throat.

6. *Sinus headache.* This headache occurs just above the eyebrows or just below the eyes. The cheekbones and the ridges above the eyes may feel sore to the touch. The person may have a stuffy or draining nose, and shaking the head or bending forward makes the headache worse.

Putting Your New Knowledge to Work for You

Find out what is giving rise to your headaches, and you can get relief by eliminating the cause. However, to be sure of yourself keep your headache record for at least two weeks. If you are still in doubt about the cause of the headaches, consult your physician. Then, begin to do the things necessary to avoid having headaches. A headache is really just a symptom or a signal that something isn't quite right. It is a message telling you to take corrective action. Beat it to the punch by preventing the headache from occurring. Some ways to do this are:

1. *Get plenty of rest each night.* If you're getting enough rest, you should wake up on your own each morning, feeling refreshed and relaxed (see Chapter 2).

2. *Have your eyes checked if you suspect you may have*

eyestrain. This is a simple but often overlooked way to get relief from headaches.

3. *Learn to get by without alcohol, tranquilizers and sleeping pills.* For headaches of the "morning after" variety, the preventative measures are obvious. Learn to relax the natural, drugless way!

4. *Try an elimination diet if you suspect food allergy.* Chapter 3 contains an elimination diet that can tell you if your headaches are due to a food allergy. By eliminating the causative food, you can eliminate the head pain.

5. *Have your sinus condition evaluated by a physician.* Sinus headaches can make you feel miserable, and the physician can offer antibiotics, allergy therapy and other medicine to control the condition.

6. *Make an effort to relax and remove tension from your life.* This is one of the hardest things to do, but it is also one of the most necessary.

How Bob B. Solved His Headache Problem in an Unexpected Way

Bob. B., a 50-year-old businessman, insisted he be seen right away. He had a severe headache, and he burst into the office and demanded something for relief: "I've had it all day, and I expect you to do something for it. And I want something that works quick."

I asked Bob to sit down, and he did. He perched rigidly on the edge of a chair. He kept rubbing the muscles at the back of his neck. I asked if he had the headaches often.

"Every day! Time I rush through breakfast and get to the store, I have one. First customer walks through the door and boom! Like somebody was choking the back of my neck. Usually aspirin makes it go away, but it didn't work today."

I wrote Bob a prescription for a mild pain reliever, but did not give it to him until he promised to return when he had more time to discuss his problem. I was sure he was having tension headaches, but I wanted him to share my diagnostic impression— and better, I wanted the patient to help in finding a way to relieve his tension.

Bob came back a week later, and we talked. He told me about his daily activities, and it was easy to see that he was building head pain right into each hour of every day. He had half a dozen employees, but never delegated authority. He always arrived at his business first, and he was the last to go home. He even worked on Sundays and holidays. He insisted on talking to every customer that had a complaint. He answered the phone; he talked to the salesmen who called on the store.

Slowly I tried to explain that by taking responsibility for everything at the store, Bob was loading himself with more tension than he could manage. Headaches were his body's way of rebelling against the excessive stress. "What you ought to do," I said jokingly, "is sell your store and let someone else have the headaches. You may not make as much money, but you'll feel better."

Bob seemed to take me seriously, and I quickly went on to say that learning to delegate authority would relieve him of much of his tension.

"Well, you've given me an idea," he said. "As long as I'm around the place I'll probably look after everything and worry like I do now. But I've got a young assistant who could manage that store. And I've been wanting to open another branch in a new shopping center. I might just try turning things over to the assistant and then keep things going slower and easier at this new store."

It was an unusual way of getting out from under a load of tension, but for Bob B. it worked!

Getting Relief from Breaking the Routine

Stress is a natural part of modern life. If your tension headaches come on about the same time every day, you may be able to prevent them by breaking the routine. Do things differently for a few days, and see if you don't free yourself of headaches. Here are some suggestions:

1. *Slow down.* Make the conscious effort, for one entire day, to slow down. Relax. Let things come to you. Go at an easier pace. Break your unbreakable schedule, and see if you don't feel better because of it! Drive more slowly. Take time to smell the flowers. Enjoy the trees, the after-

noon sky, the rich taste of fresh morning air. Listen to the music of the birds. Try very hard the entire day to let yourself be open to new sights, new tastes, new sounds.

2. *Give yourself a break.* Twice during the day, find a quiet, private place to rest. Let your body go limp. Forget about everything but resting. Think of something that makes you smile, such as what you did last weekend. Plan something pleasant for next weekend, and begin looking forward to it. Close your eyes and take a short nap. Concentrate on letting your body relax completely.

3. *Knead your tense muscles.* Rubbing tense muscles is a good way to relax them! Massage the back of your neck. Apply firm, rhythmic strokes to the painful muscles, and then lean back and let your head, neck and shoulders relax completely.

4. *Try applying heat.* If the pain persists, apply moist heat to the muscles. Use a hot water bottle or dip a wash rag in warm water and press it against the painful muscles.

5. *Avoid stimulants.* As part of your break in routine, see if you don't have fewer headaches when you cut down on coffee, tea and soft drinks. You should be able to tolerate a beverage with meals, but stimulants in between meals can add to your tension.

How Vera J. Made Use of a
Little-Known Prescription for Headache

Vera J. had headaches that were a combination of tension and eyestrain. She was a bookkeeper who worked in her home, and her problem was that she kept accounts and tried to do everything else at the same time. Just before finishing a column of figures, for example, she might have to answer the phone or the doorbell. The frequent interruptions were upsetting and brought on headaches.

I suggested that each morning and each afternoon Vera give herself a break from the tiny columns of figures. She didn't wear her glasses, and doing so was another way she could reduce eyestrain. But what she liked most was my prescription for a way to treat her headaches without drugs.

"It's used very commonly in the Orient," I told her, "and it's known as the 'pressure method.' It's especially good if your headaches are in your forehead or around the eyes. Spend about five minutes pinching the bridge of your nose or put fingers against the opposite sides of your forehead and push gently until the headache is gone. It's best if you can lie down and relax while you apply the pressure. Another way to get the same results is to lie with the crook of your arm resting across the forehead. The weight of the arm supplies the pressure, and this relieves the headache."

Vera tried the pressure method when she developed a headache, and it worked for her. Using the pressure method also took her away from her work, gave her some rest, and made her fresher when she returned to the books.

An Easy Method Barbara Used
to Have Fewer Migraine Headaches

Barbara K., a 45-year-old cosmetician, began to have spotting and irregular bleeding. A gynecologist told her she was entering the menopause. To relieve the symptoms, he prescribed hormone therapy: The Pill. The Pill did control the bleeding, but soon after Barbara began taking the medicine she began to have trouble with migraine headaches.

She had been a victim of migraine all her life, but the headaches hadn't bothered her in years. Suddenly they became so bad she had to enter the hospital. I saw her in consultation and pointed out that a worsening of migraine headaches was a well-recognized side effect of taking birth-control pills. The patient said that she'd rather have her menstrual irregularities than the attacks of migraine. We stopped the medicine, and she was able to return to work the following week.

Taking the Logical Approach to Migraine

Migraine headache is not a common cause of head pain. Many people who believe they suffer from it actually have tension headaches. Migraine is a problem that a physician must diagnose, and even the headache specialist sometimes has trouble saying for certain what is migraine and what is not. If you know you have migraine, however, take the logical approach to controlling the attacks. Follow your doctor's advice and take the medicine that has been prescribed. Remember, also, that a migraine attack can come on when things don't go right at home or at work. One of the best ways to abort an attack is to lie down in a quiet room and, if possible, go to sleep. You may be able to relax by taking a warm bath.

Separating the Minor Headache
from the One That Could Be Serious

A unique thing about migraine headaches is that they are so similar from one time to the next. Symptoms may vary from person to person, but the migraine sufferer can tell when he is about to get a headache because he has been through it before. He may have nausea or see spots before his eyes, and the headache hits him with throbbing pain on one or both sides of the head. The headache can last a few hours or a day. See a doctor if you think you have migraine attacks, and certain other kinds of headache also call for a medical exam. Here are some warning signs that mean the headache may be serious:

(1) *Headache that wakes you up each morning.* The problem could be high blood pressure. Not everyone with high blood pressure has headaches, but sometimes headache is the only symptom of this condition.

(2) *Headache with fever or vomiting.* Headache, fever and vomiting can signify meningitis or a stroke.

(3) *Headache accompanied by confusion,* pain in an eye or ear, or convulsions calls for a visit to the doctor! This is also true for headache that gets worse with straining or coughing. The headache of brain tumor is usually a dull, deep ache; the symptoms are generally worse in the morning and get better as the day wears on.

(4) *Headache following a blow to the head.* Sometimes even a seemingly minor injury can cause bleeding into the substance of the brain. The person may get up and seem alert, only to gradually lose his faculties over a period of hours or days. Always let a physician evaluate you if you develop a headache following a blow to the head.

(5) *Sudden onset of headaches in a person who has never had them before.* The onset of headaches signals that something new has happened to you. If the headache is completely different from anything you've ever had, visit a physician for a checkup.

What Medicine to Use and How to Use It

Most headache remedies contain aspirin. In fact, aspirin alone is as good as any of the combinations that contain it and other ingredients. The dosage is two five-grain tablets every three or four hours. Be sure to take the aspirin with a drink of low-fat milk or during a meal. That way, the food will help to protect your stomach from the erosive effect of the medicine. If you find that you need more than two aspirin a day, or ten in a week, visit your physician for an evaluation of the headaches.

12

How to Do Your Feet a Favor

Your feet may be one of your body's most neglected parts. They shouldn't be! Your feet are important, because you depend on them to move around and to get the exercise you need for good health. Some things you can do to avoid footache and swelling of the feet are:

1. *Wear comfortable shoes.*
2. *Give your feet the rest they need.*
3. *Take a load off your feet by losing weight if you are obese.*
4. *Reduce your intake of salt.*
5. *Control varicose veins the natural way.*
6. *Give your feet the exercise they need.*

How Clara M. Made One Change and Never Regretted It

Clara M., a 40-year-old woman, had painful feet. Like many persons of her sex, Clara put a lot of time into shopping for shoes and buying stylish, snug-fitting footwear. She paid for it by having foot pain. At the end of the day her feet would throb, and it was getting to the point where she disliked going to work more from the fear of foot pain than from any dread of the work itself. I told the patient that the treatment was simple: She had to stop wearing the tight, uncomfortable shoes she wore each day.

"But I've always worn tight shoes," Clara said. "Small feet mean a lot to me, so I buy shoes that I can barely wriggle my foot into. It's only been in the last few months that the shoes have started bothering me so much."

I suggested that Clara's foot pain had been years in the making and showed her the evidence. She had calluses on her heels and forefeet. Her toes were cramped together like cucumbers. Clara's small shoes were choking her feet and throwing them off balance so that they couldn't bear weight evenly against the ground. "Your feet aren't something just to be adorned like hair or lips or fingernails," I said. "They're a working part of your body. They deserve better care than you've been giving them."

Clara had reached the point where she was willing to do almost anything to get relief from footache. She followed my advice and bought some comfortably fitting low quarters with canvas tops and rubber soles. Her footaches stopped. She called a few weeks later to say, "I'm not ready to burn my bra, but I feel totally liberated! I just wish I had started thinking about the comfort of my feet years ago. Getting rid of those tight shoes is one change I'll never regret."

Some Little-Known Tips
You Can Use in Buying Footwear

Many people believe that you have to be uncomfortable to look good. This myth is almost as bad as the one that says small feet add to the beauty of a woman. Three thousand years ago, during the Shang dynasty, the Chinese began the deplorable act of foot-wrapping, an act that finds its modern counterpart in the woman who jams her feet into small shoes just so that her feet will appear dainty. The whole concept of desiring small feet and going to extremes to attain them is unnatural. Women have bigger feet nowadays because women are taller nowadays! The taller the woman, the bigger her feet must be to support her. But what could be more beautiful than a healthy, comfortable foot, no matter what its size?

The footwear you buy does affect the health of your feet. Here are five tips to keep in mind when selecting shoes:

Tip #1. Buy shoes that feel comfortable! Don't tell the clerk your shoe size. Let the salesperson measure your size. And don't buy shoes a size smaller than what feels good simply because the clerk tells you that the shoes

will stretch with wear. Give your feet the benefit of
the doubt, right from the start.

Tip #2. *Wait until afternoon to purchase shoes.* Your feet
collect some fluid and get slightly bigger as the day
wears on. Therefore, shoes that feel comfortable early
in the day may be too tight later that afternoon. Buy
shoes in the afternoon, when your foot is at its largest.

Tip #3. *Let the shoes fit your biggest foot.* Many people have
one foot that is bigger than the other. If you are one
of these, a shoe that fits your smallest foot may be too
snug on your opposite foot. Have the salesperson
measure both of your feet and then fit the shoe size to
your largest foot.

Tip #4. *Buy shoes with low heels.* Your heel was meant to
touch the ground during walking. Any shoe will raise
it, but high heels are most unnatural. Wearing them is
like walking on stilts; they make your ankles unsteady
and cause your toes to pinch up and ache. Avoid
these problems by choosing shoes with heels that are
less than one and a half inches high.

Tip #5. *Think ahead when buying shoes.* You have more than
one pair of shoes. Some are dress shoes, others are for
casual wear or working around the house. Think
ahead before buying shoes and wear the same socks,
stockings or anklets at the time of the purchase that
you will wear after you've bought the shoes. Casual
shoes that will be worn with thick socks may be too
tight if you were fitted for them while wearing sheer
stockings.

How Howard Learned To Reinvigorate His Feet

Howard worked in a department store as a supervisor. While
employees in his section of the store were on break, Howard filled
in for them. By the time they returned to work something else
would need Howard's attention. No wonder that his feet hurt at
the end of the day.

"You've got to get off them, give them some rest," I told
Howard. "Your feet hurt because you're mistreating them."

"But I do stop and stand still. Do that fairly often during the day. Still, my feet continue to hurt."

"Yes, but here's something you may not have thought about. Standing is harder on your feet than walking. When you're walking, one of your feet is resting while the other is bearing your weight. But standing puts pressure on both feet at the same time."

I suggested that Howard sit down for 15 minutes once in the morning and once in the afternoon. He learned to reinvigorate his feet by getting off them so that they could rest.

The Delightful Way to Enliven Your Feet

Rest is as important to the body as exercise, or eating right, or wearing comfortable shoes. Rest lets your muscles replenish their supply of energy, and it gives your circulation the time it needs to pep up your tired feet. Here are three tips to enliven your feet by giving them the rest they need:

Tip #1. Rest with your feet up on a hassock or a footstool. Slight elevation of the feet improves their circulation, and elevating your feet tends to put the rest of your body into a more comfortable position.

Tip #2. Two short rest periods are better than one long one. Getting off your feet for even a short time can do wonders! When possible, divide your rest periods into two short ones rather than one long one. And three or four rest periods are preferable to two.

Tip #3. Pull your shoes off while you rest. If possible, take your shoes off while you rest your feet. Even if the shoes fit comfortably, your tired feet will feel better unencumbered by footwear. Some people learn to kick off their shoes under the table during a coffee break, while persons working behind a desk can enjoy the delight of bare feet even while continuing to work.

How to Take the Biggest Load off Your Feet

To certain persons, the most important part of good foot care is to lose weight. Your feet must carry you, and they have to work harder when you are obese. Getting relief from aching feet is thus a good reason for losing weight. Losing weight the natural way is discussed in Chapter 6.

How Peggy W. Got Relief of Swelling by Eliminating One Thing from Her Diet

Peggy W., a 58-year-old woman, was bothered by swelling of her feet. In the morning her feet felt fine, but by supper her shoes left creases in her feet and would barely come off. My examination revealed swelling in Peggy's feet and ankles.

Many things can cause swelling of the feet, and the physician is the ideal person to diagnose the problem and recommend therapy. But Peggy's problem was not a bad heart, or kidney disease, or poor intestinal absorption of protein. Peggy's problem was that she liked salt. She used it in her cooking, she sprinkled it over her food before beginning to eat, and she chose salty foods for snacks and desserts. I estimated that she was taking in ten times more salt each day than her body actually needed. Most of the excess salt was passed out in her urine, but some of it gathered in her feet and ankles to cause swelling.

Peggy went on the low-salt diet given in Chapter 4, and within a week she no longer had swelling in her feet and ankles.

The Benefits of Using Madge T.'s Method to Control Varicose Veins

Madge T. had swelling of her feet and ankles, but the problem was not the amount of salt in her diet. The swelling persisted despite the low-salt diet, because Madge had varicose veins. The abnormal veins began during her third pregnancy and had grown steadily worse over the years.

The method Madge hit on to control her varicose veins was to wear strong elastic stockings such as those sold under the brand name SupHose®. Veins can cause swelling by oozing fluid during the day. By supporting the veins, the stockings tend to prevent swelling. Here are some tips to remember about using elastic stockings to control varicose veins:

(1) *Make sure the stockings fit your legs snugly yet comfortably.* To get the best fit, you should be measured for the

stockings by your doctor or by a person trained in fitting elastic stockings to the feet and legs.

(2) Put the stockings on first thing in the morning. The best time to apply the stockings is before you get out of bed in the morning. This way, they can keep your varicose veins from swelling with blood when you stand up. On the other hand, it's not a good idea to sleep wearing support hosiery.

(3) Wear the stockings every day. The elastic stockings do not "cure" the varicose veins. The stockings control the symptoms of the weak veins and must be worn every day to prevent swelling of the feet.

How to Give Your Feet the Conditioning They Need

Walking is good for your feet! A regular program of exercise will strengthen the bones and muscles in your feet and tone up the rest of your body as well. Here are the ways to get the most out of your walking program (see Chapters 4, 5 and 6 for other details):

- *Start slowly and then work up.* Before beginning to walk long distances, give your feet the time they need to grow stronger and healthier.

- *Wear comfortable, soft-soled shoes.* Walk in tennis shoes, jogging shoes or sandals that strap securely to your feet.

- *Walk on soft ground if possible.* A cinder hiking lane is a lovely place to walk. Plain dirt is softer than pavement, and grass is even softer. However, if you're like most people you'll have to do at least some of your walking on pavement. The exercise is worth it no matter where you do it.

- *Wear two pairs of socks.* A thin inner and a thick outer sock help to absorb foot perspiration and prevent blisters from forming. If one of your socks is an elastic support stocking, wear a thick cotton sock on the outside of it when you walk for exercise.

Common Sense Ways to Treat Common Foot Problems

The best way to treat foot problems is to avoid them. This

means wearing comfortable shoes and giving your feet the rest and exercise they need. Even so, some foot problems may arise. Here's how to treat them:

BLISTERS

Blisters occur when a shoe rubs against your foot. Accept this as a warning sign that the shoe doesn't fit properly, because even new shoes should not cause blisters. As for the blister itself, *leave it alone*. Bursting it may bring on an infection. If it breaks on its own, wash it with soap and water twice a day. It may be necessary to go without a shoe for a day or two until the blister heals.

CORNS

Think of a corn as a chronic blister. The place where it forms on your foot is a place that is continuously irritated by your shoe. The overgrowth of tough, scaling skin is nothing more than the body's way of protecting itself from injury. Use the following gentle but effective therapy for corns:

- *Soak the foot in warm water* twice a day for a week. This helps to soften the corn.

- *Apply a corn-removing chemical* after two weeks of soaking the foot. Many such medicines are on the market, but salicylic acid is the best. Ask your druggist to make up half an ounce of 5% salicylic acid in collodion. Use the wooden end of an applicator stick to apply a drop or two of this concoction to the corn. Apply the medicine after soaking and drying the foot. Cover the corn with a bandage or a small piece of cotton. Continue soaking the foot twice a day, and repeat the application of salicylic acid and collodion a week later if the corn still hasn't come off.

- *Begin immediately to prevent the formation of other corns!* The natural treatment for a corn is prevention. Wear comfortable shoes that do not press your toes together or rub the backs of your heels. A corn is a warning that your footwear has been wrong. Don't make the mistake of treating the corn without treating the *cause* of the corn!

ATHLETE'S FOOT

This fungus infection causes itching and scaling of the skin between the toes or on the bottoms of your feet. One of the best ways to prevent it is to keep the foot dry and clean. Many remedies for athlete's foot are on the market, but one of these is head and shoulders above the others. That medicine is Tinactin®. It comes as a cream in a metal tube and can be purchased without a prescription. Directions for use of Tinactin® are given on the back of the tube. Usually, one or two daily applications of the cream to even the most resistant areas of athlete's foot will produce a cure within a week. When used in the right dosage for the right condition (athlete's foot), Tinactin® is outstanding. On the other hand, if the problem on your foot continues in spite of Tinactin®, see a physician. Could be your problem is not athlete's foot.

INGROWN TOENAILS

Ingrown toenails don't usually cause a problem if you keep them neatly trimmed and wear shoes that give your toes plenty of room. An infected ingrown toenail can be serious, so visit a physician if the skin of the toes begins to swell, becomes painful or turns dark. If you are a diabetic, do not trim your toenails without first checking with your doctor.

HEALTHY FEET ARE WORTH HAVING

Healthy feet are worth having, so give yours the care they deserve. Wear soft socks or stockings, select shoes that give your feet plenty of room, and at the end of each day reward yourself with the pleasure of a good, vigorous foot massage.

13

Home Remedies for Some Common Problems

Common sense and good judgement will serve you well in treating minor illnesses. Most of the time your body will mend itself, provided you give it the chance. Backache, for example, is a most common misery. Some home remedies you can use to treat it are:

1. *Apply heat to your back.*
2. *Use aspirin for severe pain.*
3. *Sleep on a firm surface.*
4. *Protect your back from further attacks of pain.* This means a program of watching what you lift, stooping at the knees instead of bending your back, performing back exercises, and concentrating on good posture.

Rodney's Solution to His Bad Back Problem

Rodney, a 52-year-old handyman, came into the emergency room on a stretcher. He grimaced with pain when he moved and could not walk because of severe discomfort. The problem had started as a catch in his back the day before and had grown steadily worse. A spine x-ray was normal, and I diagnosed a severe back strain. I ordered medicine and told Rodney to return for another evaluation in three days. He did not return for his follow-up visit, but a few weeks later he did come in with another back strain. By this time even Rodney realized that we needed to do something to keep him from having back problems. But prevention would not be easy. Rodney owned a repair shop, and he might tear down a lawn mower one day, build cabinets the next, and overhaul a bicycle the next. He was always busy, and his work called for stooping, bending and getting into almost every position imaginable.

After Rodney could get around again, we talked about how he could protect his back from injury. One thing I stressed was that he not lift heavy objects. "Oh, I know better than to do that," the patient said. "I never lift anything heavier than this." He laughed as he reached down to pick up a piece of paper off the floor. From a standing position Rodney bent down from the waist to get the paper, and I saw his face contort with pain as he straightened up. Here, clearly, was one of the patient's problems.

"You don't have to lift something very heavy to hurt your back," I explained. "All you have to do is bend wrong, like just now when you picked up that piece of paper. Learn to save your back by stooping to pick things up. Here, let me show you." I got up and demonstrated how much easier it was to stoop down by bending the knees.

Rodney was surprised. "I never thought of that, but you're right. I do get that catch sometimes after picking up a nut or something off the floor. And as many times during the day as I have to bend down that may well be the biggest part of my problem." Indeed, Rodney stopped having backache when he learned to protect himself by stooping at the knees rather than bending his back so many times each day.

Four Steps to Overcoming Backache

You can use four steps to overcome backache. Three of these are aimed at relieving the pain of an aching back, and the fourth step is the most important one. It explains the ways in which you can keep the backache from returning.

STEP ONE: HEAT PROVIDES RELIEF!

Nothing helps an aching back like moist heat! Draw a tub of water as hot as you can stand it and ease yourself in. Stay there for 30 minutes, and you should feel better when you get out. If your back hurts too much to get into the tub, apply heat with a hot-water bottle or a thermal blanket or a rag dipped in piping hot water. Use these heat treatments two or three times a day.

STEP TWO: ASPIRIN CAN RELIEVE SEVERE PAIN

Heat will usually take the edge off the pain, but if it doesn't, aspirin is as strong a medicine as you will need. Two aspirin tablets are usually sufficient, and you should take them with no greater frequency than every three or four hours. Also, take the aspirin along with food or half a glass of liquid so that the nutrients can protect the lining of your stomach from the irritating effects of the medicine.

STEP THREE: SLEEP ON A FIRM SURFACE.

The human back is vulnerable to aches and pains, but it is also more rugged than you might think. Relaxing it on a very soft bed is not only unnecessary, it can actually harm your back. It's best to sleep on a very firm surface, and this holds doubly true if you have backache. Sometimes, almost by accident, a person will discover that a firm surface is more soothing than a soft one.

The Man Who Treated His Backache by Sleeping at the Office

Jim's office was a butcher shop, and he had worked there for so long that the smells many of us might find offensive were second nature to him. After the age of 40 he began to notice some pain in his lower back toward the end of the day. For a few years this didn't bother him very much, but one day he tried to lift an especially heavy side of beef and had sharp pains in his lower back. Because it was almost quitting time, Jim's assistant had just cleaned and covered with fresh white paper one of the large display tables at the back of the shop. Jim went moaning back to this table and climbed up on it to stretch out while his back pain went away. The firm hardwood surface felt so good that Jim soon fell asleep and did not wake up for several hours. In the following weeks, Jim began taking naps on the display table after closing time. Sometimes he reached home in time for dinner, other times not. And he complained constantly about having to sleep on the soft mattress that his wife preferred.

Jim's wife sought my help because she did not understand what was going on. I told her Jim's method of treating his backache made sense, and I went one step further by telling her how she could make the bed at home firm enough to satisfy her husband's need for back support. She bought a piece of plyboard that was ⅜ of an inch thick, had it cut so that it covered Jim's half of the bed, and inserted it between the mattress and the box-springs. Her husband was surprised and pleased by the new firmness in his mattress and no longer needed to spend the night on the wooden slab at the office.

How to Firm Up Your Own Bed

You may not need to put plyboard under your mattress if you buy the firmest "orthopedic" mattress available. However, some people with back problems sleep on a firm mattress and still put a board between it and the boxsprings. Just be sure to have the plyboard cut several inches shorter than the bed so that you can still tuck in the covers. If you are subject to back problems, sleep on a firm surface *every night.* When you are caught temporarily in a place that doesn't have a firm mattress, remember that the floor is about as hard a surface as you can find. Make yourself a pallet and let your back benefit from getting the support it needs.

STEP FOUR: PROTECT YOUR BACK FROM FURTHER ATTACKS OF PAIN

Sleeping on a firm surface helps to relieve backache, and it will also go a long way toward protecting your back from further attacks of pain. Here are some other ways to protect your back:

- *Watch what you lift.* Don't lift heavy items alone! Get help from someone else. Better yet, supervise the lifting while others do it.
- *Stoop instead of bending.* Get in the habit of bending your knees instead of your back. This way, you use your legs to do the lifting.
- *Exercise your back.* Strengthen your back muscles by doing these two exercises:
    - (1) Lie on your back with your hands at your sides. Tighten your buttocks and at the same time push up

with your shoulders. The small of your back should arch off the floor. Hold this position for a count of three and repeat the exercise several times.

(2) Lie face down, with your hands at your sides. Lift your feet and ankles off the floor and at the same time lift your head and shoulders so that your body curls up in the shape of a U. Hold the position for a count of three and repeat the exercise several times. Try to do these exercises once or twice a day.

- *Concentrate on good posture.* Keep your back's good health in mind when you walk or sit! Don't slump! Keep your shoulders back! You may find, too, that tucking a small pillow behind you will help to support your lower back when you sit. Finally, losing weight if you are obese will improve your posture and cut down on the load you're carrying around.

What to Do When You Have Fever

Fever is another common problem that you may be able to treat with home remedies. The first thing you need to do, obviously, is make sure that you *do* have fever. Obtain a thermometer and take your temperature. The average temperature taken under the tongue is 98.6° F., but your normal temperature might be a few tenths of a degree higher or lower than this. Taking a cold drink or smoking a cigarette or drinking something hot within 10 or 15 minutes before taking your temperature can lower or raise the reading. Use your judgement. If you feel feverish and the thermometer shows that you are, then it's time to do something about it. The ways to manage fever are:

1. *Record your temperature three times a day.*
2. *Use home remedies to treat mild fever.*
3. *Find out what is causing the fever.*
4. *Rest in bed and get medical help for persistent or severe fever.*

Cynthia's Method of Relieving Mild Fever

Cynthia D., a practical nurse, had flare-ups of sinusitis and often ran a fever with the episodes. Her doctor told her to call him if the fever lasted more than a day or two, and he advised her not to use aspirin to lower the fever. But Cynthia was uncomfortable even with one day of fever, and she had another way of reducing her body temperature: sponge baths. "I had helped doctors lower the temperature of sick children by giving them alcohol sponge baths, so I figured the same method would work for me. But I don't use alcohol. I just use water at room temperature. It's just as good as aspirin for lowering temperature and much quicker."

Relieving Mild Fever with the Best Treatment Possible

Aspirin, of course, is a drug well-known for its effect in lowering fever. The problem with aspirin is that it can irritate the stomach to cause nausea, vomiting or even bleeding. An alternate fever-lowering drug is Tylenol® (acetaminophen). It is available without a prescription, and the dose is one or two tablets three or four times a day. Tylenol® does not irritate the stomach, but in large doses over a long period of time it can harm the kidneys and the liver. In other words, don't make a habit of taking it, but you can safely use Tylenol® now and then. Incidentally, acetaminophen is the same drug no matter who makes it. If you find that the product made by the Bayer Company or other firm is cheaper than Tylenol®, buy it.

Alcohol or water sponge baths will lower the body temperature quickly and effectively. Still another way to get rid of fever is to place hot-water bottles filled with ice cubes on both sides of the groin and under the arms. Large arteries passing to the legs and arms absorb the coolness of the ice, and this brings down the body temperature. But the best treatment of fever is none of these methods. The best treatment for fever is to find out what is causing it and remove this cause.

Fever, after all, is a symptom. It is a reflection of something that is happening in the body. Most of the time that something is an infection such as flu or a sore throat or a cold, but fever can accompany allergic reactions, pneumonia, kidney infections, attacks of arthritis and other illnesses. The best way to relieve fever, then, is to give yourself several hours or a day to see if it will go away. If the fever continues, contact your physician.

Common Sense for the Common Cold and Flu

The common cold and the flu are caused by viruses, tend to occur most often during the winter months, and are the most common infections known. You know the symptoms: nasal stuffiness, aches and fever, sneezing, running nose, cough and an overwhelming desire to lie in bed and rest. Few would doubt that the best thing to do for a cold is to keep from getting one. Here are some ways you can do this:

#1. Stay in the best health possible! Healthy people have fewer colds than unhealthy persons. By eating right, reducing to your ideal weight, and exercising regularly, you stand far less chance of catching a cold even when the bug is making the rounds.

#2. Get plenty of vitamin C from your diet. Especially during the winter, drink orange juice or grapefruit juice every day. And eat oranges and grapefruit for breakfast or for a snack several times each week. Getting enough vitamin C will make your body stronger and more resistant to illness.

#3. Keep away from those who have colds. The best way to avoid catching a cold is to stay at arm's length from people who have one. If you are especially prone to catch colds, you may have fewer if you stay away from sporting events or movies during the peak cold months, simply because at a public event your chances of sitting close to someone with a cold are fairly high.

Chasing a Cold Away When You Get One

Take a cold seriously! Here are the things to do to get over it as quickly as possible:

#1. Go to bed for at least a day. The first day of symptoms is when your body needs rest most. Do what your natural instincts tell you. Stay in bed. By the next day you may feel like returning to your normal activities. If not, spend another day or two letting your body use all its energy to fight the cold.

#2. Get plenty of fluids. You may not feel like taking liquids, but during a cold is when you need a lot of juices, water and beverages. The fluids make your body stronger and better able to fight the infection.

#3. Take symptomatic therapy. Use an over-the-counter decongestant for stuffy or running nose and take aspirin for fever, aches or the "blah" feeling that goes with a cold. For cough, you can buy a remedy or make your own at home. A good one that is available without a prescription is Robitussin-DM®. It contains the drug dextromethorphan, which has the effect of reducing the severity of the cough. Use this drug only as directed on the label and do not take it unless your cough is very troublesome. Some people prefer to use homemade cough remedies. Try taking a teaspoon or two of honey with a few drops of lemon juice in it. The honey will form a soothing layer over the irritated lining of your throat. You can use it as often as you wish to treat your cough.

Three Ways to Overcome Nagging Mouth Ulcers

A shallow ulcer that appears suddenly in the mouth and lasts for a week or two can be a painful nuisance. It hurts when you eat, bothers you when you talk, and nags you the rest of the time. These sores are known as canker sores, and their cause is not known. Nor has a cure been found, but you can use the following three methods to get relief from the ulcers:

1. *Use a mouth wash three times daily.* Select a pleasant-tasting mouth wash and rinse your mouth thoroughly with it three times a day. This helps to remove the dead flesh that can build up around the ulcer.

2. *Apply a local anesthetic to the ulcer.* Nupercainal® is a topical anesthetic that is available without prescription. Apply a small amount of this anesthetic directly to the ulcer (you'll need the help of a mirror). Repeat the treatment three times a day. Many people find that the best time for application of Nupercainal® is just before eating, so that food and drink won't cause the ulcer to burn during the meal. Be cautious about using Nupercainal® if you're sub-

ject to skin allergies, because this medicine can provoke an allergic reaction.

3. *Coat the ulcer with Tincture of Benzoin®.* Tincture of Benzoin® is available without prescription. Athletes sometimes paint it on the soles of their feet as a "foot toughener," and nurses use it after surgery to help tape stick to the patient's skin to hold the surgical dressing in place. Dip the cotton-tipped end of an applicator stick in the benzoin and apply the brownish liquid lightly to your mouth ulcer. (Again, you'll need the aid of a mirror or an assistant.) Rinse your mouth vigorously with water after the treatment, because benzoin left in your mouth could stain the teeth brown. The benzoin works by covering the nerve endings of the mouth ulcer. You can use it several times a day, and if applied before meals it will keep the ulcer from burning while you eat. Another medicine that can coat the ulcer is Gly-Oxide®. You can buy this mixture of peroxide and glycerol without a prescription. Apply it directly from the container to get half an hour or more of relief from pain. It is recommended for use after meals and at bedtime.

Some people have fewer ulcers by eliminating chocolate, spicy or abrasive foods, and nuts from their diet. Perhaps the best preventive is to avoid chewing gum.

14

How to Look and Feel
Your Best Every Day

The Greeks had a saying for it: *Mens sana in corpore sano:* a
healthy mind in a healthy body. How you think and react to things
does affect the way you feel! You may have known people with apparently healthy bodies who were very unhappy. On the opposite
side of the coin are persons with severe illnesses who manage
despite the affliction to radiate an inner joy that is enviable. It is
true that we are slaves to our feelings and moods, but it is also true
that controlling these moods is possible. To look and feel your best
every day, you need to:

One: *Believe in yourself!*
Two: *Speak your own mind!*
Three: *Talk out your problems with others!*
Four: *Fill your life with happy things!*
Five: *Make good health a part of your life!*

Harry O.'s Secret for Sales Success

Harry O. was one of the top salesmen for a well-known insurance company. Everyone spoke highly of this man and of the
amazing sales record he had compiled in his 20 years with the company. Harry gave sales seminars, and I had a chance to hear him
speak. I was disappointed with the salesman's introductory com-
ments. He shared the opening session with several dull speakers
and didn't seem all that dynamic himself. How could he be the top

salesman for this entire region? I asked myself. I determined to talk to him and got my chance during a coffee break.

"As a matter of fact," Harry told me, "I take a low-keyed approach. Other salesmen—and especially the sales managers—are always setting impossible goals of so many sales a day, and it makes the men feel like they're starting off behind, almost knowing they can't get there, so what the heck. Well, that kind of feeling is one of the worst things for a salesman. What you need out there in the territory is confidence. Any success I've had is due to taking the opposite tact. I try to go out in the morning and make just one sale. I tell myself that if I do make that one sale I won't starve to death, which is true. Then, with one under my belt, I say heck, 'Why not another?' "

As he spoke, Harry's eyes began to burn brightly with enthusiasm. His face took on a glow of confidence; he seemed to grow taller. "Once the ice is broken for the day," he continued, "I can relax. The rest of my sales come easy, because I'm under absolutely no pressure. I'd just about as soon sit there and talk about baseball or anything else the prospect wants to talk about as discuss insurance, and when the customer senses I'm not pressuring him it makes him trust me."

"If you could list the one thing that's been your key to success, what would it be?"

"I'm glad you asked," he said with a smile, "because that's going to be the topic of the next session of our seminar." About five minutes later the second session began. Harry walked silently to the blackboard and wrote his secret for all to see. Everyone in the audience sat spellbound for the next hour and a half, and all came away with a good feeling for having attended. The three words that Harry wrote on the blackboard and spent the time discussing were "BELIEVE IN YOURSELF!"

Try This One-Minute Pause
That Can Refresh and Invigorate You

Taking measure of your own abilities and worth as a human being can be a refreshing experience. We live in a world that seems filled with negative, sad or heartbreaking events. Without a conscious effort on your part, these negative events can turn your thoughts in that direction. You have but to read a newspaper or watch the TV news to see what I mean! To counteract the negative things that can influence your thinking, you have to be positive and self-confident. You have to be able to give yourself pep talks, to turn your thoughts to pleasant things, to focus on what you can do rather than what you can't do. Believing in yourself is the best way to achieve a positive, self-confident personality. Every time you feel depressed or begin to doubt your own abilities, try this one-minute pause that can refresh and invigorate you. First, find a quiet place where you can be by yourself. It can be anywhere, but some place out-of-doors or with a view to the outside is preferable. During this one minute, do three things:

#1. *Picture a vast, deep cliff and mentally pitch your problems over its edge.* Say goodbye and good riddance to them as they fall away from you! Feel unshackled? You should!

#2. *Think of something good that you have done for someone else within the last day.* Plan something good for someone else. Doing for others is a positive act that has a magical way of reinforcing your own sense of self-worth.

#3. *Tell yourself that right now, this very moment, you are an okay person.* Draw strength from your knowlege that your life counts for something in the world! You have helped others, you have contributed, and you will continue to do these things. There's nothing wrong with patting yourself on the back! Believe in yourself, and you can replace doubt and fear with a surge of happiness and a sense of well-being! Feel the tension leaving your body?

I suggest you write these three steps down on an index card and carry them with you. When you feel the need, take the one-minute pause and reap its benefits. You can take this refreshing pause as often as you like, but I recommend it like medicine: three or four times daily as needed for refreshment.

How Liz Did One Thing and Changed Her Entire Life

Liz M. was a 40-year-old woman who worked alongside 20 or 30 other people in a large office building. Liz wanted very much to be popular with her co-workers, yet achieved just the opposite. She always butted in, talked louder than the others, and seemed genuinely programmed to make enemies. Virtually everyone in the office had felt the wrath of her tongue or been the subject of one of her deflating remarks. Believe me, these are not the tools one uses to build popularity, yet it came as a shock to me one day when Liz blurted out that she didn't understand why no one liked her.

Trying not to hurt her feelings, I asked her how much she really liked herself. She said, "If you took a misery count I'd score 100%, so it must not be much."

I suggested that Liz's problem might be that since she didn't like herself, she might unconsciously be treating others as if they didn't like her. It turned out that Liz had been brought up to believe that vanity of any kind was wrong. She was taught to wear plain clothes, to dress without attention to her hair or face, and to take a supporting role in the things she did. All her life she had fought against this training, and because she was intelligent she was able to be a leader more often than a follower. At the same time, down deep, she still doubted her own worth as a human being. I gave her a pep talk on the benefits she could derive from believing in herself and had her repeat the one-minute pause every hour on the hour throughout the day. The results were nothing less than miraculous. Once Liz started liking and believing in herself, she had no need to put others down. She found that when she treated people fairly they treated her the same way. She became one of the most popular people in that office, but she found something that was more important to her. She found the inner contentment she had been searching for.

Taking Your Place in the World by Speaking Your Own Mind

You have things to say. Say them! Believing in yourself and speaking your own mind go hand in hand. Even before Liz learned to believe in herself she was able to give her opinion about almost everything you could mention. In fact, she was too willing to give her opinions, and this was one of her problems. Speaking out about everything is not what I mean by speaking your mind, but giving your honest opinion when you are asked for it is a healthy act. Speaking up helps to rid you of doubt and insecurity. Your opinion is as good as the next person's, and your speaking up may give others the courage to do so.

The Woman Whose Courage Changed
a Cloud of Smoke to Clean, Fresh Air

A few years ago the CBS-TV affiliate in Austin, Texas featured the story of a woman who worked at the State Health Department. This woman did not smoke and was offended by the clouds of cigarette smoke that continuously drifted past her desk. (Yes, I said that she worked at the State *Health* Department.)

Finally this lady worked up her courage and complained to a supervisor about the amount of smoke that was polluting her environment. The supervisor reacted by firing her! This happened on a Friday afternoon and was no doubt a stunning blow to the woman's ego. However, because she believed in herself and in what she had spoken out about, she did not give up. She obtained the services of an attorney, and by the following Monday morning she had her job back. The TV cameras zoomed in on several men who were moving the lady's desk to a less smoky area of the building.

Precisely because of people like this woman, state office buildings, schools and many other public buildings now carry signs that forbid smoking except in designated areas. A small ripple can sometimes create a tidal wave.

Solving Problems by Talking
Them Out with Someone Else

Believing in yourself and speaking your own mind are two things that will help you look and feel your best every day. Good mental health depends on another ingredient as well: You need to have someone with whom you can talk out your problems. This is what friendship is about. You see, each person has problems. His happiness depends on how he reacts to the problems. Hearing your troubles, another person may be able to offer solutions you haven't thought of.

Darlene's Discovery of a Way to Be Happy

Darlene, a middle-aged widow, was unhappy for many reasons. She was lonesome and in a rut. She rarely went out, she knew that life was passing her by, and yet she seemed unable to do anything about it. Luckily Darlene had a friend, Judy, who took her along to a weekly discussion group held by several women.

As Judy told it, the women had been meeting informally for several months. They had coffee and talked. One woman would tell of a problem, and the others would answer. The only rule for the sessions was that the women be completely honest with one another. Darlene said not a word at the first meeting, but did express an interest in returning the following week. Judy took her. About the third or fourth meeting, Darlene began to speak, and soon her inner turmoils were boiling out for all to hear. Her husband had been killed in an accident, and she blamed herself for not being killed along with him. She had planned to accompany him to the game, but changed her mind at the last minute. Her husband left alone and not ten minutes later was dead from a head-on collision. This had happened five years before. Since then, Darlene had made an effort to forget the past. But she was still reminded of her husband each time she went home, each time she saw their old friends, each time she went to work—for she was still employed by the same firm where they had both worked. She couldn't escape the visible reminders that her husband was dead and that sadness had entered her life.

One of the women in the group said, "Darlene, what you need to do is get things going again! Change your life! Why, I don't see how you've lasted five years doing what you're doing. Get out of that house! Find a different job! Go on a trip! Start over!"

Tears filled Darlene's eyes. She said, "I've thought of doing those things. But . . . but I don't want to do them because I think it wouldn't be fair to the memory of my dead husband."

"Fair?" another woman said. "Fair? He'd want you to do what's fair to you! Your years together were wonderful, but they're over. Your husband is dead. Now it's up to you to make a new life for yourself."

Several other women agreed. The next week Darlene did not return to the group. The participants worried about her, because they weren't sure how she had taken their suggestions. However, a week later Judy got a letter from Darlene. Darlene wrote: "I wanted so much to come back to tell you how much I appreciated what you and your friends did for me. But I just couldn't wait to get away from those things once I realized the truth of what you said. I'm in Florida now, apartment hunting. In a few days I'll be back to pack my things. It wasn't necessary to quit the company. I've arranged a transfer to Miami. I'm deliriously happy about this chance for a new start, and as soon as I get situated, the first thing I'm going to do is start a discussion group just like the one you wonderful people have going."

A discussion group isn't the only way of talking your problems out. All you need is one other person. It may be your spouse, a good friend, your neighbor or a close relative. The important thing is to find someone with whom you can be open and honest. And let the other person talk that way to you. Problem solving works in two directions.

How to Fill Your Life with Happy Things

Believe in yourself and think about the good things in life! Make the conscious effort to put some pleasure into your life. Every day! Here are some suggestions:

#1. Plan fun into your activities. Each morning, as you plan the day's activities, reserve some time for enjoyable events. You may want to look forward to dining out that evening or to visiting a friend or relative. Your daily walk may be what you enjoy most. Think about these pleasant things and plan your day around them.

#2. Do something special for yourself. Every few days, at least once a week, do something special for yourself. Take an afternoon off. See a movie. Play golf. Bowl. Eat out. Go for a long drive. Do something special, and do it for the sheer pleasure that doing it gives you!

#3. Put music into your life. The French actor Louis Jourdan, best known for his role in the musical "Gigi," said, "The bitterest disappointments in life are almost completely dissolved by one hour of good music." Maybe you like classical music, or maybe you prefer to hear the twang of a guitar. Find a radio station that plays your kind of music and surround yourself with this pleasant atmosphere.

#4. Relax and take things in stride. Take the one-minute pause that will refresh and invigorate you! Or make it a

ten-minute pause. Build break periods into your routine, even if you are working for yourself. You may find it relaxing to go outside (or inside) or to sit and listen to the world around you. Give yourself some quiet at least once a day, and here is a way to tell if your environment is quiet enough for you to let loose your tensions and relax. You're in a quiet place if, when you take a drink of carbonated beverage, you can hear the effervescence of all those carbon dioxide bubbles exploding inside your mouth. It is a whispery hiss like the rise and fall of waves on a distant shore, a marvelous and relaxing sound! If you've never heard it, you may not know how much quiet you've been missing.

The Clean-Living Way to a Long and Happy Life

A healthy mind in a healthy body means that you can't have one without the other, but it also means that having one *will help you get the other.* Thus, everything you do to have better physical health makes it easier for you to live without tension and worry. Good health is cause for happiness! And the more you believe in yourself and appreciate your own worth, the more you will strive to take pride in your body and give it the care it needs. A good mental outlook will make you want to:

- *Stop smoking (or not start).*
- *Refrain from using unneeded drugs (including alcohol).*
- *Reduce to your ideal body weight and stay that way.*
- *Get started on a daily program of exercise.*
- *Eat the foods that will give you good health.*
- *Avoid the foods that can contribute to high blood pressure or heart disease.*
- *Drink enough water to keep your kidneys healthy and your bowels efficient.*
- *Get the rest that you need every day.*

In other words, the clean-living way to a long and happy life is built upon the sound principles of good health that are discussed in this book.

To Your Good Health and Longevity

It seems that every animal species has an upper limit to its life span. A dog can live 20 years, a chicken 30 years, a horse 50 years. But a human being can live 110 years or longer. The mystery is not so much that a life span of 110 years is possible, but that so few people attain great longevity. One man who had reached the age of 103 was asked if he would do anything different if he had to live his life over. "Yes," the man said. "If I'd known I was going to live so long, I'd have taken better care of myself." His answer was tongue in cheek, because taking care of yourself *is* the secret of longevity.

You can hold on to your youth and live longer than average by following the steps in this book. Having good health will do more than just extend your life. You'll feel happier and get more out of life than the person who is waylaid by frequent illnesses. The important thing is not so much the information in this book, for to be quite honest, you could find many of these same health tips in other books. The vital thing is that you understand that you are the only one who can give yourself good health. Too many people for too long have expected this precious gift to come from a magic tonic or a sure-fire remedy or some other gimmick. It doesn't work that way. You have to do the work and make the sacrifices to have good health, but on the other hand, you are the one who stands to benefit most. You, and the ones you love.

It won't be easy. Nothing good ever is. But it can be done, and *you can do it.* Begin by returning to the Contents of this book. Mark the parts that have special meaning for you. Then, read these pages again and begin putting the advice to work in your life. Make lists. Put up notes to yourself. Keep a ledger of your progress. Plan each day, each week and each year to do what it takes to have good health! Make exercise, sensible eating and getting plenty of rest a part of your life. Practice makes perfect; your goal should be nothing less than making healthy living a lifetime habit.

I wish you every success.

Average Desirable Weights for Adult Women
Wearing Indoor Clothing and No Shoes

HEIGHT*	SMALL FRAME	MEDIUM FRAME	LARGE FRAME
4'8"	95	102	112
4'9"	98	104	114
4'10"	100	107	118
4'11"	103	111	121
5'0"	106	114	124
5'1"	109	117	127
5'2"	112	120	130
5'3"	115	123	133
5'4"	119	127	137
5'5"	122	131	141
5'6"	126	135	145
5'7"	130	139	149
5'8"	134	143	153
5'9"	138	147	158
5'10"	142	151	162
5'11"	146	155	166
6'0"	150	160	172

*If your height does not come out at an even inch, take an average between the weight given for the preceding inch and the next higher one. For instance, if you are a medium-framed woman and your height is 5'4½", your ideal weight is the average of 127 (the weight given for 5'4") and 131 (the weight given for 5'5"), or *129 pounds*.

For information on predicting your frame size, see the note beneath the chart of ideal weights for men.

Average Desirable Weights for Adult Men
Wearing Indoor Clothing and No Shoes

HEIGHT	SMALL FRAME*	MEDIUM FRAME	LARGE FRAME
5'1"	114	122	132
5'2"	117	125	135
5'3"	120	128	138
5'4"	123	131	141
5'5"	127	135	146
5'6"	130	138	149
5'7"	134	142	154
5'8"	138	146	158
5'9"	142	150	162
5'10"	146	155	166
5'11"	150	159	171
6'0"	154	164	176
6'1"	159	168	181
6'2"	163	173	186
6'3"	167	178	191
6'4"	172	183	196

*Your frame is your bony structure. If you don't know whether you are big-boned, small-boned or in between, your doctor can give you an estimate. However, you can predict your frame size by looking at the width of your wrists, fingers and feet. If these structures are large, your frame is large. But if your hands and feet are small, your frame is too. Most people fall somewhere in the middle, in the medium range.

Index

A

Activities:
  blood-building, 19
  inactivity causes constipation, 130
  new activities to give energy, 31
  secret of youth, 97
Alcohol, 93, 134, 149-150
Allergy:
  to antiperspirant, 141
  to aspirin, 145
  cause of headache, 149
  to cosmetics, 142
  to feminine hygiene sprays, 141-142
  to food, 50-52
  to Nupercainal, 171
  to poison ivy, 142-144
  of skin, 138-139, 141
American soldiers, autopsy reports, 73
Anemia:
  aplastic, 27
  G-6-PD deficiency as cause of, 27
  infections as cause of, 29
  iron deficiency, 21-25
Angina pectoris, 80

Antacids:
  Gelusil, 132
  Maalox, 132
  for relief of gas, 131
  to relieve heartburn, 131
  Riopan, 132
  Trisogel, 132
Arthritis:
  bony arthritis, 102, 105, 115
  calcium growth, 108
  claims of "cure," 116
  combining heat and exercise, 108
  five ways to get relief, 101
  importance of weight loss, 115
  "Monday arthritis," 111
  osteoarthritis, 102, 105, 115
  rest as treatment, 109
  rheumatoid, 104
  use of aspirin, 112
  use of heat, 102-105
  value of exercise, 106
  value of rest, 110
"Arthritis pain formula," 112
Aspirin:
  allergy, 145
  cause of anemia, 27

187

Aspirin *(cont'd.)*
  dosage, 114
  for fever, 169
  for headache, 147, 155
  one form as good as another, 113
  relief from arthritis, 112
  relief from backache, 166
  side effects, 114, 135
Athlete's foot, 163
Austin, Texas, 177
Average desirable weights, 182, 183

B

Backache:
  four steps to overcoming it, 165
  how to avoid it, 167
  sleep to prevent it, 166
Bakeries (use of shortening), 79
Baking versus frying, 81
Belching, 130
Believe in yourself, 174
Birdwatching, 36, 102
Bladder infections, 120
Blood:
  amount pumped by heart, 82
  bleeding, causes of, 24-25
  bleeding ulcer, 133
  effects of exercise on, 29, 83
  foods that build blood, 21
  how to build rich blood, 19-30
  red blood cells, 24
  in the stool, 26
Blood pressure:
  dangers of high blood pressure, 53
  diastolic pressure, 59, 69-70
  drugs vs. low-salt diet, 55
  elevation from drugs, 41
  headache a symptom, 154
  how to take your own, 69-70
  keeping a record of it, 70
  lowering it by exercise, 35
  natural ways to lower it, 53-69
  sphygmomanometer, 69-70
  systolic pressure, 59, 69-70
Bones, 115
Bowel movements:
  constipation from Gelusil, 132
  enema, 129
  normal frequency, 127

Bowel movements *(cont'd.)*
  position for, 128
  regular habit, 128
  time to spend, 128
  walking aids normality, 130
Bracelet (medical identification), 146
Burow's soaks, 144

C

California, 96, 143, 146
Calories:
  in beer, 93
  burned in exercising, 97-98
  burning to lose weight, 96
  in carbohydrate, 43, 47, 90
  in desserts, 92-93
  in fats, 90
  in fruits, 92
  in proteins, 90
  in snack foods, 93
Cancer, 24, 45, 94, 154
Cane, use by arthritics, 112
Canker sores, 171
Carbohydrates:
  calorie content, 43, 47, 90
  food content, 78
Cereal, whole grain, 21
Chemicals:
  antimalarials, 27
  aspirin, 27 (*see also* Aspirin)
  blood-damaging, 26-28
  drugs (*see* Drugs)
Chicago, 81
Cholesterol:
  cause of heart attack, 43
  eggs' content, 21, 43, 77
  in juicy steak, 43
  less in high-quality ground beef, 79
  low cholesterol diet, 78
Cigarettes (*see* Smoking)
Circulation:
  bad effects of smoking, 67
  better with exercise, 83, 85-86, 159
  heat increases, 102
Citrus fruits, 23, 52, 121
Coffee, 41, 134
Colon:
  irritable colon, 135
  spastic colon, 135

Colorado, 29, 81-82, 138
Common cold, 169
Constipation, 126, 129-130, 132
Cooking sensibly, 80
Coronary disease, 73
Cosmetics:
  cold cream, 139
  hypoallergenic cosmetics, 142

D

Death:
  due to heart disease, 73
  suicide, 39
Denver, Colorado, 29-30
Diabetes:
  "cure" from losing weight, 48-50
  exercise helps, 85
  prevention by losing weight, 37
  trimming toenails, 163
Diarrhea:
  due to colchicine therapy, 46-47
  due to food allergy, 50
  from irritable colon, 135
  from Maalox, 132
  usually self-limiting, 136
Diet:
  elimination diet for food allergy, 50-52
  for irritable colon, 135
  for kidney failure, 123
  low cholesterol, 78
  low-fat to help heart, 74-81
  low-salt dangerous in kidney disease, 125
  low-salt for blood pressure control, 55
  for quick weight loss, 95
  six-feedings to lose weight, 95-96
  to treat diarrhea, 136
  for ulcer, 133-135
Dreams, 38-39
Drugged sleep, 38-39
Drugs:
  acetaminophen, 169
  acetylsalicylic acid, 113
  adrenalin, 145
  Alpha-Keri, 140, 144
  aminopyrine, 27-28
  amphotericin B, 122
  antacids (*see* Antacids)
  aspirin (*see* Aspirin)
  barbiturates, 39

Drugs *(cont'd.)*
  Benadryl, 144
  calamine lotion, 144
  chloramphenicol, 27
  colchicine, 46-47
  colymycin, 122
  dextromethorphan, 171
  Domeboro tablets, 144
  gentamicin, 122
  Gly-Oxide, 172
  gold salts, 122
  iodides, 145
  kanamycin, 122
  laxatives (*see* Laxatives)
  Lubath, 140
  narcotics, 145
  neomycin, 122
  nitrofurantoin, 27
  Nivea, 140
  not the only treatment for
    arthritis, 102
  Nupercainal, 171
  penicillin, 145
  phenacetin, 113, 122
  phenylbutazone, 27
  polymyxin B, 122
  PreSun, 139
  propylthiouracil, 27
  Robitussin-DM, 171
  sleeping pills, 38, 149-150
  sodium salicylate, 114
  steroid hormones, 145
  stimulants (speed), 41
  streptomycin, 122
  sulfa drugs, 27
  sunscreen, 139
  Tetracycline, 145
  that can harm blood, 27
  that can harm kidneys, 122
  The Pill, 153
  thiazides, 55
  Tinactin, 163
  Tincture of Benzoin, 172
  tranquilizers, 149-150
  Tylenol, 169
  vancomycin, 122

E

Eating:
  to avoid food allergies, 50-52

Eating *(cont'd.)*
  to avoid ulcer, 134
  for better health, 42-52
  to build the blood, 21-23
  to help the heart, 74-81
  to lose weight, 90-96
Enema, 129
Energy:
  doesn't come from breakfast, 44-45
  fat is stored energy, 90
  how to have more, 31-41
  20-minute refresher, 98
Esophagus, 132
Exercise:
  abdominal, 63, 130
  blood-building potential, 29, 83
  to build the blood, 29, 83
  cycling, 60
  definition of, 60
  exercycle, 98
  foot wear, 64, 161
  to give energy, 31, 33-36
  to improve the lungs, 83
  jogging, 60, 85
  to lower blood pressure, 35, 58-65
  range of motion, 106
  to relieve constipation, 130
  secret of youth, 99
  start slowly, 63, 161
  to strengthen the back, 167
  to strengthen the heart, 83
  stretching exercises, 63
  swimming, 60, 97, 109, 111
  types of 60, 97, 161, 167
  warm-up, 63

                    F

Fat:
  bakeries cook with animal fats, 79
  calories in, 43, 47, 90
  cutting fat off meat, 80
  fatty drippings from meat, 81
  food content of, 78
  number calories in one pound, 90
  saturated, 21, 43, 74
  unsaturated, 74
  ways to eat less, 74-81
Fatigue, 31, 109, 148-149
Feet:
  athlete's foot, 162

Feet *(cont'd.)*
  blisters, 162
  corns, 162
  exercise will help, 161
  foot-wrapping, 157
  how to enliven them, 159
  ingrown toenails, 163
  myth about small feet, 157
  support hosiery, 160
  tips on buying shoes, 157
Feminine hygiene sprays, 141
Fever, 168-169
Florida, 143, 178
Flouride, 26
Food allergies, 50-52, 144, 149
Food and Drug Administration, 45
Foods:
  beans, 46, 75
  better health from, 42-52
  bologna, 79
  bread, 42, 77, 96, 136
  butter, 75
  buttermilk, 74-75
  cereal, 42, 44-45, 77
  cheese, 42, 75, 136
  cinnamon, 52
  corn, 52
  corn oil, 75, 81
  cranberry juice, 121
  cream of rice, 77
  cream of wheat, 77
  doughnuts, 91-92
  eggs, 21, 43, 77, 136, 144
  egg substitute, 78
  fish, 45-46, 57
  food colors, 45, 52
  frankfurters, 45, 79
  fruit juice, 78, 118, 121, 123, 170
  fruits, 42, 45, 47, 58, 79, 91, 123,
      129, 170
  gravy, 52, 81
  ham, 43, 57, 77
  ice cream, 42, 75, 136
  iron-containing, 21
  liver, 21
  liverwurst, 79
  margarine, 42, 75
  Mazola oleo, 51
  meat (*see* Meat)
  Melba toast, 93
  milk (*see* Milk)
  natural ones are best, 45

Foods *(cont'd.)*
 oatmeal, 77
 pastrami, 79
 pea family, 52
 peanut butter, 45, 79, 136
 pie, 47, 79
 potato chips, 45, 56-57
 potatoes, 81, 129
 poultry, 46, 79, 136
 rice, 46, 129, 136
 salami, 45
 sausage, 43, 57, 77
 sausage substitute, 78
 sherbert, 51
 strawberries, 79, 144
 tomato, 52
 vegetables, 23, 42, 45, 58, 129
 wheat germ, 45, 47, 129
Fried foods, 81

G

Gallbladder trouble, 92
Gas, 130
Gastritis, 114
Glasses, 148
Gout, 46-47

H

Happy things, 179
Headache:
 could be serious, 154
 due to eyestrain, 148
 due to The Pill, 153
 from hangover, 149
 "headache record," 148
 migraine, 153
 most frequent causes, 148-149
 "pressure method" to treat, 153
 symptom of brain tumor, 154
 tension headache, 148, 150-153
Heart:
 fantastic pump, 82
 gets more rest with exercise, 87
 heartbeat causes blood pressure, 69
Heart disease:
 angina pectoris, 80
 congestive failure, 22, 31, 82
 is due to many things, 72-73, 76

Heart disease *(cont'd.)*
 myocarditis, 82
 prevention best treatment, 73
 smoking as cause, 86-87
 woman's risk, 73-74
Heat treatment:
 for backache, 165
 by electric blanket, 103
 heating pad, 103
 from hot bath, 103
 lamp, 103
 moist heat, 103-104
 protecting the skin, 103
 to relax tense muscles, 152
 use in arthritis, 103
High heels, 158
Honey (cough remedy), 171
"Honeymoon cystitis," 120

I

Infection:
 of bladder, 120
 cause of fatigue, 31
 sinusitis, 29, 149, 169
Insect bites, 141
Insomnia, 38
Intestinal flu, 136
Iron:
 deficiency, 21
 foods rich in, 21
 iron tablets, 26
 loss in menstrual periods, 23, 25
Itching:
 from dry skin, 139-140
 home remedies for, 143-144
 "itch-scratch cycle," 140
 from poison ivy, 142-144

J

Jogging, 60, 85, 97
Joints, 106, 115
Jourdan, Louis, 179
Journal of the Amer. Med. Assoc., 96

K

Kidneys:
 damage from phenacetin, 113

Kidneys *(cont'd.)*
   drug-induced damage, 113, 122, 169
   failure, 124
   importance of check-up, 124
   kidney stones, 119-122
Korean War, 73

                              L

Lactase deficiency, 50-51
Lactose, 51
Laxatives:
   affect entire system, 129
   food laxatives, 129
   how to break the habit, 126-127
   how to reduce the dose, 127-128
Longevity, 87, 181
Louisiana, 105

                              M

Marbling in steak, 80
Mattress (firm for back), 167
Meat:
   best iron source, 21
   food group, 42
   lean meat best, 43, 45
   reduce intake for kidney disease, 123
   reducing fat content, 79-81
Medical check-up:
   after an injury, 146, 154
   before starting exercise program, 62, 83
   for cause of anemia, 24
   for cause of headache, 149, 154-155
   for fever, 169
   for food allergy, 50
   for foot problems, 163
   for heartburn, 132
   for kidney disease, 125
   for migraine headache, 153
Meningitis, 154
Menopause, 153
Methylene blue, 118
Mexico City, 29-30
Miami, Florida, 29-30, 179
Milk:
   cause of allergy, 50-51
   food group, 42
   high-salt food, 56

Milk *(cont'd.)*
   ice milk, 75
   low-fat milk best, 48, 74
   milk sugar, 51
   source of saturated fat, 74
   to wash aspirin down, 114-115
Mineral oil, 104

                              N

Natural ways to control blood
   pressure, 53-70
Natural ways to normal
   digestion, 126-136
Natural ways to relieve headache, 147-155
New Orleans, 29

                              O

Obesity:
   cause of footache, 159-160
   danger signal, 49
   losing weight for more energy, 36-37
   recognizing cause, 90
Olive oil, 140
One-minute pause, 174
Orient, 153

                              P

Paraffin, 102, 104
Peptic esophagitis, 131-132
Petrolatum jelly, 104, 139
Physical therapist, 140
Pillow, use in arthritis, 112
Poison ivy, 142-144
Poison sumac, 142-144
Pope Innocent VIII, 19
Protein:
   calorie content, 43, 90
   food content, 78

                              R

Range of motion exercises:
   benefits of, 106-108
   ones to perform, 107-108
Reducing (*see* Weight loss)

Reflexes for bowel, 127
Relaxation:
before taking your blood pressure, 70
to music before sleeping, 40
to prevent headache, 151-152
way to have more energy, 31
way to lower blood pressure, 66-67
Renal papillary necrosis, 113
Rest:
get the amount you need, 41
to prevent footache, 159
to prevent headache, 149
to relieve a cold, 170
to treat arthritis, 110
Reward program, 99
Rheumatologist, 106

S

Salt:
danger of excessive intake, 54-55, 160
high content in processed foods, 56-58
high-salt foods, 56
low-salt antacid, 132
low-salt foods, 57
Shang dynasty, 157
Sinusitis:
cause of anemia, 29
cause of fever, 169
cause of headache, 149-150
Skin:
correct technique for drying, 138
dry skin and itching, 140
hives, 144
"itch-scratch cycle," 140
keep it young and alive, 137-146
oils for dry skin, 140
rash due to food allergy, 50
soaks to treat rash, 143-144
treatment for rash, 143-144
wrinkles, 137-138
Sleep:
amount you need, 41
choice of bed, 40
drugged, 39
good sleep habits, 39
to help arthritis, 110
normal rhythms, 38
Smoking:
cause of heart disease, 86-87

Smoking (*cont'd.*)
cause of lung cancer, 86
effect on blood flow to legs, 67
effect on blood pressure, 67-68
increases stomach acid, 135
Soaks:
for arthritis, 103-104
for corns, 162
for skin rash, 143-144
Soap:
allergies to, 142
"antibacterial," 137
to protect against poison
ivy, 143
use mildest possible, 137
Soda (soft drink):
calorie content, 48, 93
coke as example, 93
as water substitute, 118
Speak your mind, 177
Sphygmomanometer, 69, 70
Steak, 21, 43, 46, 80, 124
Stethoscope, 69-70
Stimulants, 41
Stooping instead of bending, 165
Stress:
cause of headache, 151-152
how to handle it, 66-67
Sugar, 94
Sun, cause of skin damage, 138-139
Sunscreens, 139
Suntan, 138
Sweetening, 94
Swelling:
of the feet and ankles, 37, 82
relief from low-salt diet, 160

T

Talk your problems out, 177
Tea, 41, 118
Temperature, oral, 168
Texas, 143, 177
Thyroid:
disease of, 31, 88
disease not a cause of obesity, 89
hormone, 88-89
Tiredness (*see* Fatigue)

U

Ulcer:
  bleeding from, 25, 133
  complications, 133
  duodenal, 133
  effect of vitamin C on, 122
  of mouth, 171
  stomach, 114
Urine:
  antiseptics, 120-122
  blue color from drug, 118
  flushing action, 120
  product of kidneys, 117
  what yellow color means, 119

V

Varicose veins, 37, 85, 160
Vitamins:
  folic acid, 23
  in low-fat milk, 75
  vitamin B$_{12}$, 23
  vitamin C, 23, 135, 170
  vitamin D, 75, 139
  vitamin E, 75

W

Walking:
  distance to go, 84-85
  to help arthritis, 109, 111
  to help feet, 161
  how fast, 84
  how to turn it into fun, 64
  lets feet rest, 159
  number calories burned, 97
  program to build the heart, 84
  to relieve constipation, 130
  value of short walks, 61
  what to wear, 64

Water:
  best medicine for bowels, 128
  as cause of skin dryness, 140
  drinking it helps kidneys, 120
  healthy drink, 47, 122
  hot water for arthritis
    relief, 103-104
  how much to drink, 118
  least expensive medicine, 118
  limits to how much in
    kidney disease, 123
  to wash aspirin down, 114
Weight loss:
  average desirable weight, men, 183
  average desirable weight, women, 182
  be your own best friend, 100
  creates a change, 93
  drug therapy, 41
  to have more energy, 31, 36-37
  to help arthritis, 115
  helps feet, 159-160
  to help the back, 168
  how exercise helps, 83
  importance of staying thin, 95
  to relieve heartburn, 131
  seven tips, 90-96
  three ways to achieve it, 89
  from walking, 97
Weight Watchers, 37
Whipped topping, non-dairy, 79
Whirlpool baths, 140
Wisconsin, 76

Z

Zero weight gain as goal, 99
Zinc oxide, 139